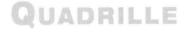

QUADRILLE

how to do

everything

and still have

time for
yourself

dawna walter

Publishing Director: Anne Furniss
Consultant Art Director: Helen Lewis
Project Editor: Nicki Marshall
Designer & Illustrator: Coralie Bickford-Smith
Production Controller: Beverley Richardson
Special Photography: Andrew Wood
Picture Researcher: Nadine Bazar
Picture Assistant: Sarah Airey

First published in 2001 by
Quadrille Publishing Limited
Alhambra House
27–31 Charing Cross Road
London WC2H 0LS

This edition first published in 2004.
This book previously appeared under the title
New Leaf, New Life.

British Library Cataloguing-in-Publication Data
A catalogue record for this book is available from
the British Library.

ISBN 1 84400 075 3

Printed in China

contents

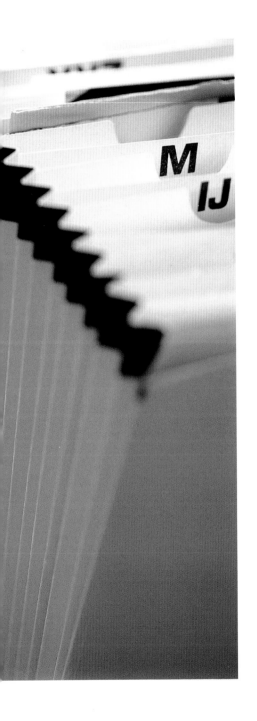

introduction 6

rise and shine 8

getting around 26

nine to five 44

homework 56

sanctuary 78

entertaining 94

relaxation 124

bedtime 138

suppliers and further information 152

index 158

acknowledgements 160

introduction

" Just for today, do not worry. Just for today, do not anger. Honour your parents, teachers and elders. Earn your living honestly. Show gratitude for everything. "

DR MIKAO USULI, *The Ethical Principles of Reiki*

We're here for a good time not a long time, right? Simply put, life is far too short to spend it being unhappy. That's not to say that each day of our lives is spent in perfect bliss, but it is most certainly something to strive for, isn't it?

We all go through periods in our lives when we start to assess our lifestyle. It happens when things seem out of control, or when we reach a significant birthday. Life events such as the passing on of a loved one, marriage or the birth of a child are often a catalyst for making us sit down and assess our values. Even the start of a new year can give us the determination to change the things in our lives that do not make us happy and develop a programme of personal goals to get us on the right track.

To set the record straight, I am by no means perfect. My life can, and does, get out of control. Papers stack up. I don't always clean my refrigerator and I sometimes hide things in cupboards so I don't have to deal with them. I lose my temper more often than I would like and I do have days when my house is not the sanctuary that I would like it to be. But I do practise what I preach, and when things are not looking acceptably clean or tidy, perhaps once every couple of weeks, I have a cathartic purge and tackle the areas that seem to have got the best of me. One step at a time, as they say in many self-help programmes.

How to do Everything and Still Have Time for Yourself is about making a fresh start. It is about making the most of the things in life that we must do, and creating more time for those things that we want to do. It is about trying to create balance and about having some fun in the process.

The first thing that is needed to effect change in your life is the will to change it. Make up your mind to do it and you will. It really is as simple as that. Remember that it takes six weeks of doing anything to make it a habit. What is six weeks in the grand scale of life?

The second thing that you need is an open mind. Be receptive to new ideas. Listen to your intuition. We all have a little voice telling us the right thing to do. Call it coincidence or spiritual help from above. Trust it. You'll find that the more open you are to the things around you, the more you'll believe in yourself. Try new things. Don't be afraid to fail. Nothing ventured is nothing gained. Make it a point to try and learn something new each day. Expand your thinking and your life will certainly be more interesting.

Look after yourself, both emotionally and physically. Many holistic therapies attribute the causes of major disease to emotional blockages in our body. Think about it. Take it on board. We only have one body for the duration and we want it to last a long time. Keeping things inside emotionally is a major cause of stress and can lead to heart disorders and gastric problems. Let it out in a constructive manner.

Sing more – in the shower or on the way to work. Sing in the car or listening to your favourite tunes. It doesn't matter if you can't carry a tune. It really does release some pent-up emotion, as any good country and western song will bear witness.

Try some meditation to clear the mind and gain perspective. There is nothing mystical about it. Just sit in a quiet place for 15 minutes and concentrate on your breathing. As a thought enters your mind, imagine big, fluffy clouds floating by and place the thought on the cloud to return to later. Practice makes perfect. Give it a go.

Think about the things you eat. Let's face it, if you don't eat fat, it's unlikely that you'll get fat. Eat more fresh vegetables and whole grains. You don't have to become a vegetarian to be healthy – just limit your consumption of meat and fat obtained from animal sources. Stay away from processed foods like shop-bought meals and cakes. Simple carbohydrates such as sugar, honey, white flour and alcohol are absorbed rapidly into your system, which causes your body to secrete insulin to lower your blood sugar levels. This makes it more likely that your body will convert calories into body fat. As we all know – you are what you eat.

Physical exercise of any kind will keep stress at bay. It is essential for both emotional and physical wellbeing. Find the right programme for you and fit it into your daily routine. Walk to work. Do a class in the gym. Practise yoga at home. Do tummy crunches when you get up in the morning or before you go to bed at night. Remember, after six weeks, it will be a part of your life.

Each day, be grateful for the things you have. Make a point of finding five things that happened during the day that you are grateful for. It can be as simple as someone smiling at you when you are walking down the street. Be thankful and you will feel less bitter about the things that you think you don't have and more appreciative of the nice things that do happen each and every day that can often be taken for granted. Be more generous – this doesn't have to involve money. Say thank you whenever someone has done something nice. It will dramatically change the relationships that you have with those around you. Try it and see.

Your home is your personal retreat. It should be the place where you can recharge your batteries and relax and enjoy being with your friends and family. Many of the things that we need to do to keep it running smoothly are nothing more than acquired skills. We are not all born perfect housekeepers, but there are many time-saving tricks of the trade to enable you to spend less time doing the drudgery and more time relaxing. Learn how to share responsibilities with those you live with and feel more content. You only have to get your home organised once for it to become much more manageable to maintain. Start today and in no time it will be your sanctuary.

There is no time like the present. It is a gift. Have fun with it. Take control of your life. All you have to do is turn over a new leaf and you'll discover a new life. Make it happen. If you have the determination, the way forward will be simple. Start now.

How to do Everything and Still Have Time for Yourself is about making a fresh start. It is about making the most of the things in life that we must do, and creating more time for those things that we want to do.

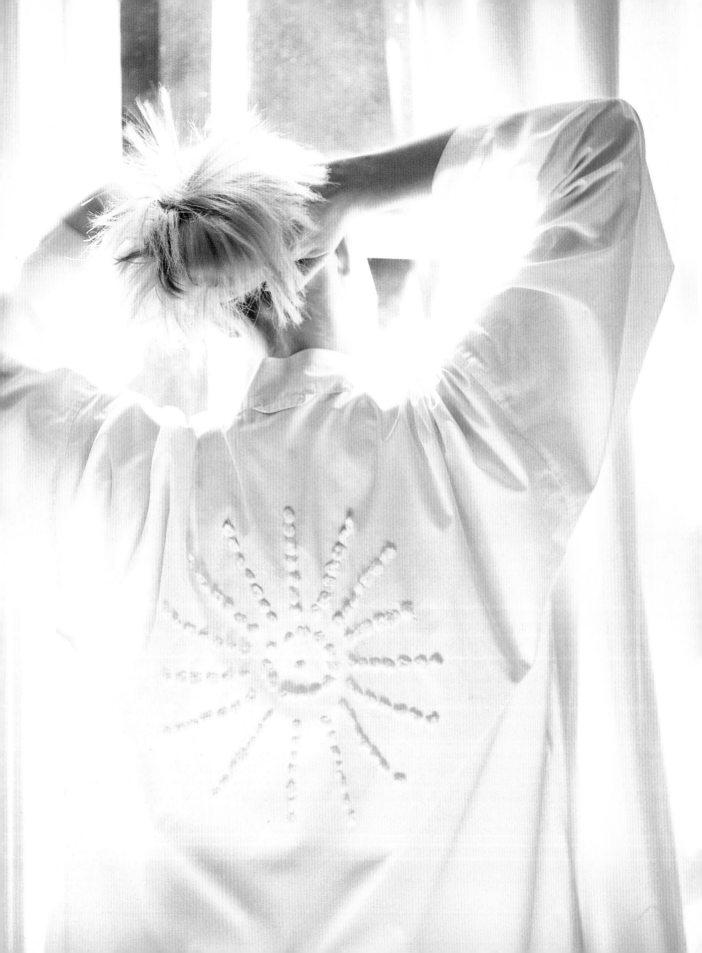

rise and shine

"The past is history. Tomorrow is a mystery. Today is a gift.

That is why it is called the present." ANON.

Each day brings with it the promise of a new beginning. Wake up ready to make the most of every minute. Open your eyes and look around you. See the morning light. Enjoy the moment. Seize the day. Rise and truly shine.

How you wake up in the morning determines what you accomplish during the day. Think about it. If you have overslept the panic sets in as you race around the house trying to catch up with yourself; your day goes from bad to worse as you have to squeeze more things into less time.

Be in control of each new day. Know what you need and where to get it. Relax. Take care of your body. Take time in the bathroom. Enjoy the process. Invigorate yourself in the shower.

Save time. Clear out your wardrobe. Make space for the things that you really use. Develop a 'uniform' to limit the indecision of what to wear. It doesn't have to be boring: a few basics and key accessories can produce a number of different combinations for any occasion.

Make sure you have the essentials in your bathroom: the shampoo should be within reach and clean towels waiting for when you step out of the shower. Your bathroom time is precious: use it to luxuriate before a hectic day and make it a pleasurable experience.

Leave the bedroom and bathroom as you would like to see them when you return. There is nothing worse than an unmade bed or clothes strewn across the floor when you are ready to retreat

for a peaceful evening. It only takes a few minutes. Make it a habit.

Most importantly, schedule some time to sit and have your morning coffee or tea. And don't forget that breakfast is the most important meal of the day. Don't leave your house with an empty tummy – you need the energy.

Gather your thoughts. Make a list of what you hope to achieve during the day. Think about the things you didn't accomplish yesterday and why you were unable to get them done. Do them first thing today.

Today is a present. This is its beauty; you never know what it contains until it has been revealed. No matter what it holds, embrace it with enthusiasm. Go on, make your day.

up, up and away

Sleep is the body's way of recharging, but too much sleep, like too little, can leave you lacking the energy required to embrace the day with a positive attitude. Cramming every minute of the day with activities, even with a good night's sleep, can make you still feel fatigued when you wake up.

We are creatures of habit. Our bodies become accustomed to the sleep patterns and routines that we develop over the years. If getting up in the morning fills you with dread, try a little mind over matter to break the cycle. If you think you can change things, you can.

Feeling overwhelmed can arise from not having time to relax. If you think that you are constantly doing things every minute, the feeling of not having enough hours in the day overwhelms you the moment you arise.

Rather than thinking that you need more sleep to feel refreshed, you might be surprised to find that an hour's less sleep can give you the personal time you need to relax and do things that you never seem to find the time to do. Enjoy a quiet cup of coffee without the phone ringing or members of your family requiring your attention. Read the morning paper. Go for a jog. Take an extra 10 minutes in the bath. Be selfish. Think about yourself for once with no pressures or demands on your time. It will make a difference. Practice makes perfect.

What you see when you open your eyes in the morning can affect your mood for the day. Sunlight streaming through a window gives you a sense of wellbeing. A sense of order in the things around you gives you a feeling of being in control. Always take the time in the evening to make sure that the things around you are left as you would like to see them in the morning. Start the day with a feeling of calm and optimism and you will make the most of your day.

Every now and then, shake things up a little: you don't want to be predictable, do you? Paint the walls in your bedroom a completely different colour. See if it changes your attitude. Move around all the furniture in your room and gain a different perspective. Have a lie-in. Get up to watch the sunrise. Change your routine. Burn some essential oils to clear the way: grapefruit is uplifting; sage is for clarity. Get all the help that you can.

Be thankful every morning to be alive. Take a few minutes before you get out of bed to think about the things in your life that make you happy. Be grateful for all the things you have. Think about the goals you want to achieve and remember that there is every chance you will achieve them if you remain determined to succeed. Accentuate the positive and eliminate the negative. Try it. Think about it during the day. Smile more often. Pay attention to what a difference it makes!

Plan your day, but don't set it in concrete. Things happen. Be flexible. Go with the flow. Learn something new each day. Learn from your mistakes. Set your mind to achieving your goals and focus your energy on the job at hand. Get into it. Do the best that you can. Be kind to yourself. And never forget that tomorrow is another day.

Accentuate the positive and eliminate the negative. Try it. Think about it during the day.

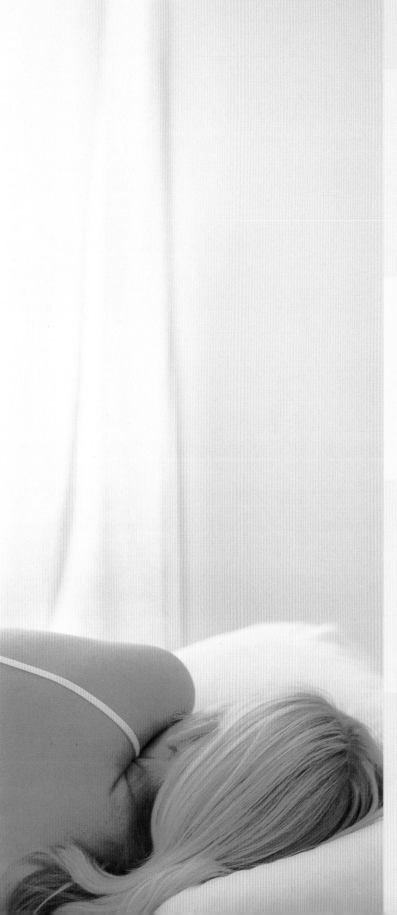

10 ways to save time in the morning

...so you can stay in bed longer or, better still, get up and enjoy those extra few minutes.

Wash your hair the night before.

Lay out your clothes for the next day before you undress at night.

Don't iron in the morning.

Get your breakfast things ready before you go to bed.

Don't leave any dirty dishes in the sink from the night before.

Colour-code your wardrobe. It really does help.

Organise your underwear drawer so that you can find things quickly.

Gather everything you need to take with you in one place.

Always keep your keys in the same place.

Do one job today that you have on your list to do tomorrow.

10 ways to have a healthy day

Stretch your mind and refresh your body at the start of the day and give yourself a head start.

1

Meditate for 15 minutes

Close your eyes. Breathe in slowly and exhale slowly, feeling your tummy deflate. Imagine your thoughts floating away on fluffy, clouds. Gain insight and relax.

2

Drink it all in

Drink a large glass of mineral water to help detoxify. Remember to do this throughout the day. It helps to keep your appetite at bay while cleansing your system.

3

Get the power

Take a power shower and exfoliate all of your dry skin. Stimulate your circulatory system with a sponge and concentrate on all those areas where fat cells seem to congregate. Finish with cool water and wake up those extremities.

4

Feel fruity

Breakfast is the most important meal of the day but it doesn't have to be heavy. Try squeezing some fresh juices or make a smoothie using no-fat yoghurt, ice cubes and a selection of your favourite fruits. Stick them in the blender and shake, rattle and roll.

5

Vital vitamins

If you want to ensure that your body receives all the vitamins and minerals it requires or you would like a vitamin boost to fight off a cold or reduce hayfever symptoms, supplements may be the answer. Go to your local chemist or health food store and ask their advice on the best vitamins for you. As with all remedies, check with your doctor if you have any medical conditions.

6

Fat-free

Pay attention to the amount of fat in all the food you eat. It will astound you. The healthiest diet consists of no more than 10 per cent fat or about 20–25g of fat per day.

Try to choose foods that consist of no more than 3g of fat per serving. The best foods are vegetables, fruit, whole grains, beans and non-fat dairy products. It's as simple as that!

7

De-caffeinate

Limit your consumption of caffeine, which is found in coffee, tea, chocolate and soft drinks. Cut your intake throughout the day and relax. Try herbal teas, decaffeinated coffee, mineral water and fresh juices. Notice the difference.

8

Sweet enough

Simple carbohydrates like sugar, white flour and alcohol cause your body to secrete insulin to lower your blood sugar levels. The body will then be more likely to convert calories into body fat. Limit your consumption of sugar and see if there is a change in your body fat.

9

Walk on the wild side

Start your day with a brisk 20-minute walk. Use your arms and increase your heart rate. Wear the proper trainers to cushion the impact.

10

Feel the burn

Start your day at the gym. Take a class. Swim. Use the machines. Mix it up so that it doesn't become boring. Your outlook on the day will change dramatically.

bathroom blitz

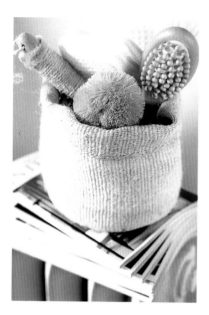

For me, the perfect bathroom has an abundance of light, a fabulous bath and a powerful shower, a stack of freshly laundered towels and a collection of deliciously scented soaps and candles. Bliss. Make your bathroom a place where you enjoy spending time.

Take the time

A calm and organised bathroom can be a wonderful place to relax and gather your thoughts: a place to cleanse not only your body but also your soul. One of the most personal rooms in your house, it says a lot about your priorities. If your bathroom is a haven of relaxation you enjoy the process of grooming and presenting yourself to the world. What does it say about your life if your appearance means nothing to you?

Use your space

Because bathrooms are usually the smallest room in your house, you need to think of creative ways to keep your things together. Try tall, thin shelving units that can fit in the tiniest of spaces or shelving that fits over the toilet.

Sensory appeal

Make your bathroom appealing to the senses. Filled with great scents and textures it will be intimate and cosy. Baskets are a great way to keep your essentials grouped together and come in so many colours and shapes that you can find the perfect one for almost any

use. I have a number in my bathroom and each one is filled with all the things I need for my grooming regime. I can quickly find anything I need and all the clutter is kept at bay.

Close to hand

When in your bathing area you should have everything you need within close reach. Make sure you always have enough shampoo and soap nearby. Clean towels should be on hand as you step out of the bath or shower and your bathrobe should be accessible but in a location where it can keep dry.

Soft and gentle

Indulge in your favourite products to refresh and invigorate you. Give your head a massage when shampooing. Apply conditioner to your hair and keep it on long enough for it to work. Always use moisturiser when you finish bathing – put it on while your body is still slightly damp and it will lock in the moisture.

Repeat performance

Before you leave the bathroom, quickly wipe out the residual soap and water from the bath or shower. It will make it a nicer experience when you use it next time. Hang your wet towels up to dry. Always put the caps back on anything you've used and check that the soap is not sitting in water. Make sure that you haven't run out of anything; if you have, buy it today.

bathroom buddies

Start your day with a little help from your bathroom buddies. Here are the essentials to make the experience a delight.

Power shower
Invigorate. Stimulate. Breathe in the steam. Get a fresh, clean start on the day.

Wake up!

Large bath towels
Keep them warmed. Make sure they are soft. Give yourself a good rub-down.

Get your energy flowing.

Slippers
Get off on the right footing. Don't slip and slide.

Selection of aromatherapy bath products
Get a little help to start your day. Stimulate your senses. Awaken your mind.

Moisturiser
Take the time. Nourish your skin. Lock in the moisture while your skin is still damp.

Good lighting
Always see yourself in the best light.

Calm down. Know what you need. Always have choices.

Your favourite bathrobe
Always keep it hanging around for when you might need it.

A huge mirror
Always look at yourself straight in the eyes. Like what you see. Face the day.

putting on your face

Clean your bathroom mirror. Take a good look at yourself. Your skin tells the story of your life.

If you haven't been taking care of yourself, you will know it immediately. Pay attention to the signs. You know the cause of it. Drink less. Get more rest. Eat better. Relax.

Let the sunshine in. If you put your make-up on in the sunlight you will have a truer picture of what it looks like and it will work well in most lighting. If you don't have a naturally bright, sunny space, fake it with artificial lighting.

Morning make-up rituals should begin with a clean face. If you have thoroughly cleansed the night before and your face isn't shiny, wash with warm water and then moisturise. If you have slightly oily skin, use your favourite cleaning products and then rinse thoroughly before moisturising.

Accentuate the positive

Less is more. For an everyday look, you shouldn't have to spend more than five minutes applying your make-up. Enhance your best features and play down your weaker ones – it's an obvious make-up rule but it really does work. Younger women with a good, even complexion can get away with the bare minimum – a touch of foundation, lipstick or gloss and defined brows. Older women should think about concealer if they develop dark shadows around the eyes and nose.

Only your hairdresser knows for sure

Different hair colours may require a different emphasis of features, so if you are thinking of experimenting with a new look then remember that your make-up may have to change too.

In general, circles or shadows under the eyes are more visible on brunettes, but in turn brunettes may not require mascara or eyebrow definition. Most blondes could benefit from extra definition around the eyes and brows, particularly if their hair is very light. Redheads may need to define their lips so that their glorious hair does not overshadow their facial features.

Tricks of the trade

Professional make-up artists all agree that neutral shades of make-up are the easiest to apply and will effectively enhance your natural beauty. Powders are much easier to use than creams or pencils as they are easier to blend. Use a foundation/powder compact for an easy, light covering or, even better, use a tinted moisturiser with sun protection. To define the eyes use a dark eye shadow, either wet or dry, applied with an eyeliner brush. To define your brows, use an eye shadow colour slightly darker than your brow and apply lightly with a hard-edged brush.

Use a neutral lip liner several shades darker than your lips to outline them. This can be used with all shades of lipstick and should never stand out, so feather it instead of drawing a hard line. Lip liner is also a great way to stop lipstick from bleeding.

The best way to keep lipstick in place is to use a base coat of good lip balm and let it dry. Apply your lipstick over the top of this and then blot with tissue. Build up a few layers of lipstick, blotting in between each, until you put on the final layer. It really does work.

Powder blush should be applied with a proper, full-sized brush to alleviate that streaky look. Go for the 'just kissed by the sun' colour. To set your make-up, use loose powder and a big fluffy brush, but make sure that your powder doesn't make you look too pale.

Putting on the ritz

When you are going out for the night, give your face special attention, but don't overdo it. Treat yourself and the evening will have more meaning. Take the time to remove your daytime make-up and moisturise. Relax on the bed for five minutes while the moisturiser seeps in. Close your eyes and listen to your breathing. Apply your make-up using slightly richer or brighter tones than for your daytime look, but remember – less is more. Give your hair a lift. Spray your favourite perfume into the air and enter the scent.

Take a good look at your fabulous self in the mirror. If you feel good you will look good.

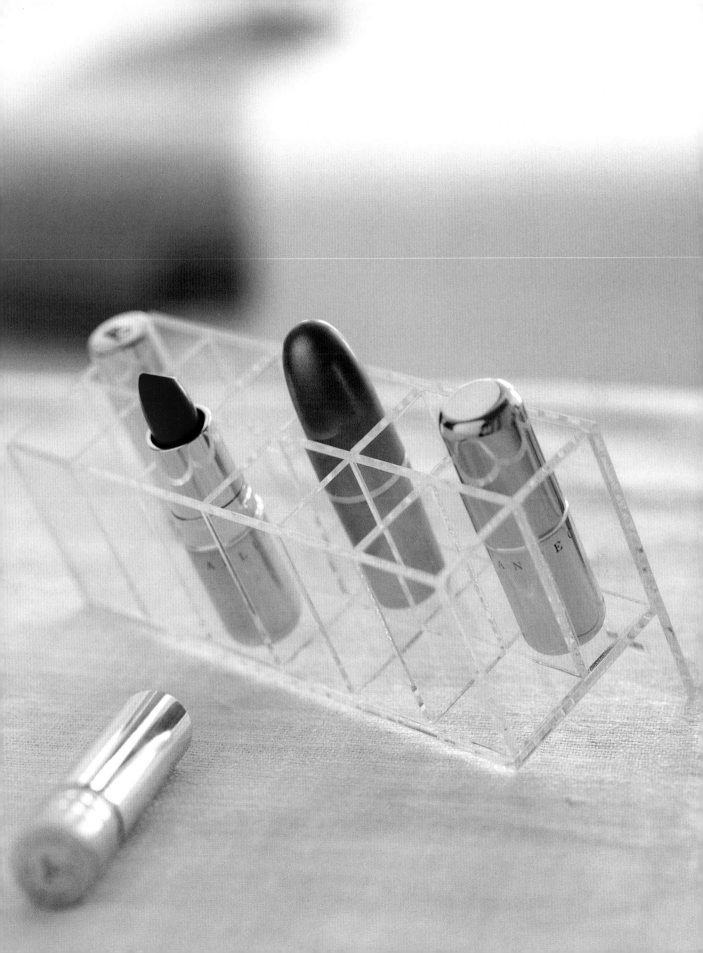

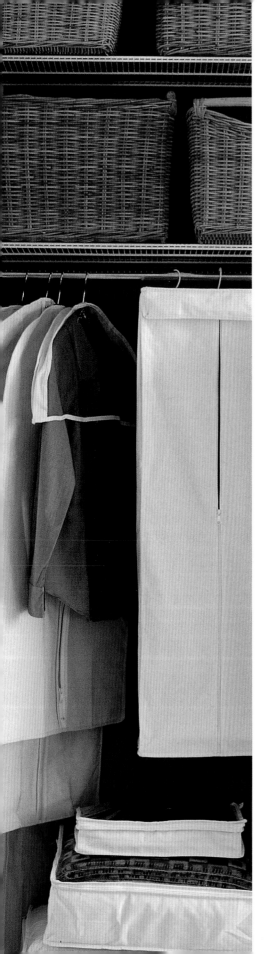

organising your wardrobe

Truth or dare

The truth is that you just can't fit another thing into your over-stuffed wardrobe. There are three layers of clothing on every hanger and you can never find what you want to wear when you want to wear it.

The dare is to admit that there are things in your wardrobe that haven't seen the light of day for years. You have even forgotten what clothes you have because it's been so long since you saw them all. It's time for a purge.

Honesty is the best policy

You may need to have someone to help you sort through your wardrobe who will tell you the truth. Get your best mate round – they may walk away with a few of your goodies and will love the chance to relive your past with you.

Make it fun – have a laugh. A weekend afternoon is an ideal time to get the project done. Put on some great tunes – reggae does it for me – pour yourself a glass of wine, or whatever puts you in the mood, and get going.

Out of the closet

Do not be embarrassed by what you uncover even if you find things that have been lurking in your closet for10 years without being worn. Your cast-offs can go to charity and make you feel

better about gaining the weight, buying on impulse or making the World's Worst Dressed list. It will also give both of you the chance to remember who you once were and to be thankful that you have moved on and changed, hopefully, for the better!

Pile it up

Get a good supply of bin liners. You will need them. Everything must come out. Sort the clothes into four separate piles – see what's hot, what's not (opposite). Be honest, or the whole exercise will have been pointless. Take your time to decide properly as you'll have to live with the consequences.

Remember that phrase about clouds and silver linings? It will all be fine in the end. You will save so much time every day that the pain and agony of all this organising will fade quickly.

Clean slate

Once you have been through all your clothes, you will know how many items need to go back into the wardrobe. Some of these might need to be cleaned first. If you get anything dry-cleaned, remember to remove the plastic bags from the dry-cleaner's before you hang the clothes up, as they don't allow your clothing to breathe and can yellow fine, light-coloured fabrics.

what's hot,
what's not

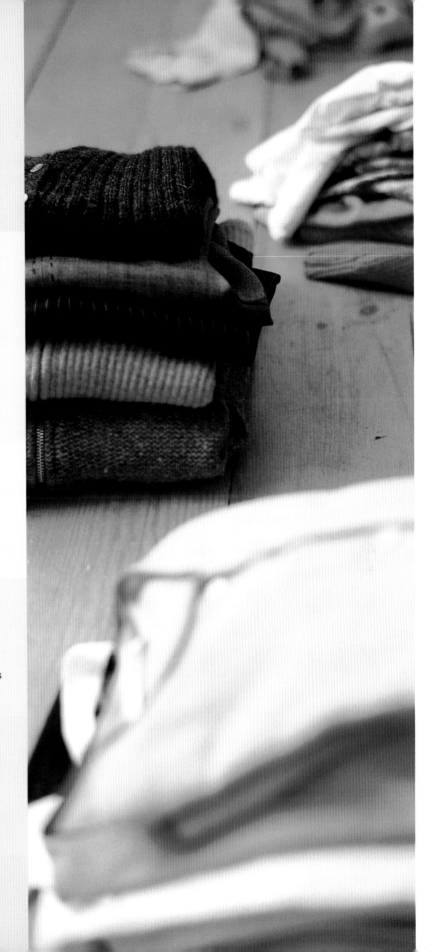

Pile One – On the go team
- Anything with a stain that can't be removed.
- Anything that is ripped or torn. Unless you repair today, give it up.
- Anything that is way too small. You know the truth.
- Anything that you haven't worn in a year.

Pile Two – Sentimental journey
- Anything that you really can't bear to part with but you never wear. These clothes will be stored in a less accessible location.

Pile Three – Here and now
- This is your working wardrobe. These are the things that you wear every day. Put your hand to your heart and make sure that this is the truth.

Pile Four – To everything there is a season
- These are clothes that you wore during the last season and you will wear when the weather changes.

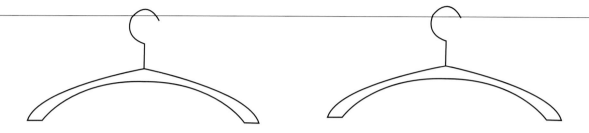

The end is near

Now that all your clothes have been placed into one of the four piles, you need to start putting them away. Start with your short hanging things at one end and continue graduating down in length, with your longest garments at the opposite end. You are going to put like with like – group your shirts, suits, trousers, skirts, dresses and long things together, by colour. Although it may sound slightly neurotic, it really does make sense and will help to keep things ordered in the long run.

The truth about hangers

Hangers really make a difference. Wire hangers destroy the shape of your clothes. Any hanger of the wrong size or shape can ruin the shoulders of a garment and make it look old before its time. Hangers come in different shapes for different clothing. Broad-shouldered hangers are good for suits and coats of medium to heavy fabrics. I prefer wood, as it never bows and the lightweight versions are ideal for dresses and shirts. And remember – there is a difference between men's and women's hangers. Size counts.

Bars and clips are the way to hang trousers and skirts. Try to look for grips that have a rubber surface. They keep creases out and stop things slipping. If you are truly strapped for hanging space, multiple hangers can hold five times as many garments. Make sure you have some cedar wood in your wardrobe, preferably as hangers. Moths hate the scent. If the cedar fragrance starts to fade, revive it quickly by lightly sanding the wood with fine sandpaper.

Control yourself

You are now in the driver's seat. You know exactly what you own and where to find it.

Take a step back and have a good look at everything. We are, after all, creatures of habit. So you have 10 white shirts. Will you buy another? Are you buying variations on the same theme each time you shop? Now that you can see everything together, you also know which addition to your wardrobe would make the most impact. You will save yourself money.

You will also find that you have created lots of space under your short hanging clothing. This is a great place to stack your shoes, in their boxes with a photo attached, on a stacking shoe rack or in plastic drawers. Don't forget to keep them clean and well heeled – they tell people a lot about you. You can also use this space to house a small chest of drawers to hold your folded clothes. All the same principles apply. Like with like, by colour. You'll find things in a trice.

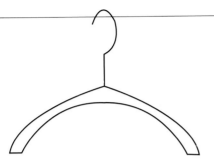
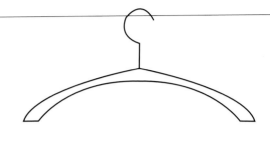

It was worth it, wasn't it?

Back to the beginning. Offer anything in the Go Team pile to your friend. If you are not likely to have a jumble sale in the near future you have two choices. The first is the feel-good factor. Put the bags in your car now and take them to your closest charity shop. It really does make you feel good. Anything in top condition could be taken to a Designer Resale shop to generate a bit of extra cash or, if you prefer, you could give these clothes to charity, too.

Out-of-season clothing needs to be carefully packed away, labelled and placed in a less accessible location: under your bed, in the loft, under those awkward stairs or above your wardrobe. If you travel throughout the year to different climates, keep a core range of out-of-season clothing in with your current clothes so that you can pack in a hurry without stress.

Make sure that all of your out-of-season clothing is laundered before you put it away, as moths thrive on dead skin and leftover particles of food.

When you unpack your clothes later on, you don't want to have to spend time cleaning and pressing them again, so fold with care.

The ideal container is something that breathes, like canvas. Cardboard will be a possible second choice, but plastic is not really suitable. Place cedar blocks or lavender sachets amongst the clothes to keep them smelling sweet and to repel insects. Label the outside of each container clearly with a big luggage tag so that it will be much easier for you to find the things you need and to swap over your clothes whenever the season changes.

Now for those sentimental things. When was the last time you really looked at them? If you have something very precious or beautiful, think about putting it on display. Hang a hook on your wall and make it a decoration for your bedroom. If it isn't worthy of display, pack it away in acid-free tissue inside a linen chest or an extra suitcase. Don't forget about it or it isn't worth keeping.

Reward yourself

Give yourself a big pat on the back. You have risen to the occasion and you are now in control. You will save yourself loads of time each day and feel less frustrated.

Indulge yourself. Have a hot fudge sundae. Take a very long bath. Put your feet up and read a book. You only have to do this twice a year.

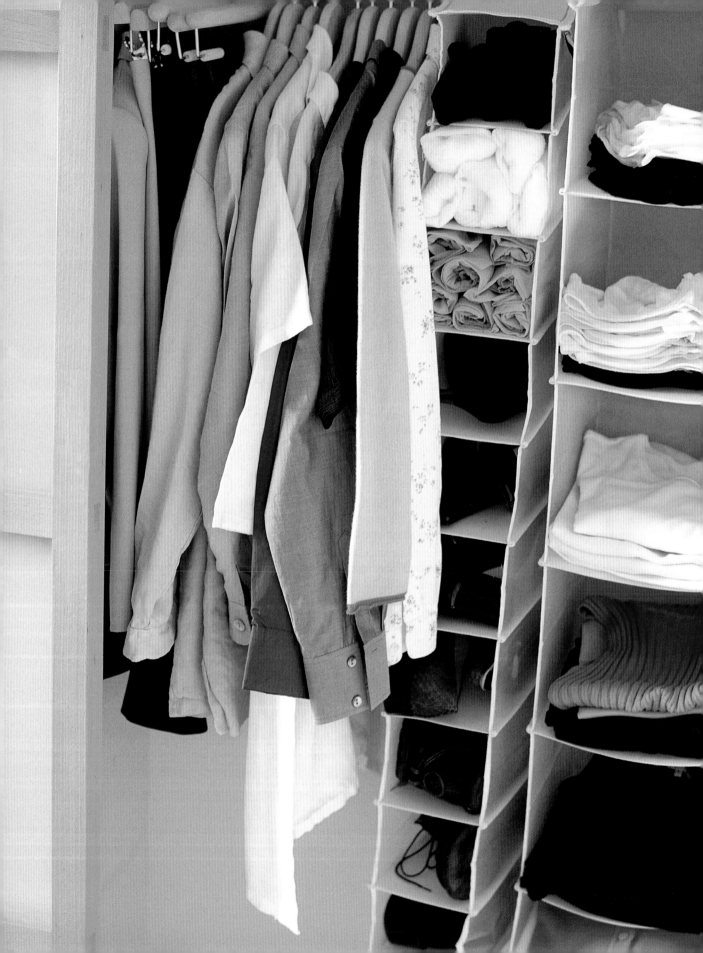

the look

We wear 20 per cent of our clothes 80 per cent of the time. The old stand-bys that you are drawn to on a late morning are the clothes that take little time to put together. You know what I mean. You look good and feel good with minimal fuss. Go with your instincts. Figure out what you really like and why. Be decisive. Pay attention to how you look and how you feel. Have a good look in the mirror and like what you see.

The uniform

Go to your wardrobe and take out the 20 per cent that you wear most often. You will instantly know what they are. Think about the reasons that these are your favourites. Are your choices based on colour, type of clothing, shape or fabric? Whatever the elements are that make certain items work for you, remember them the next time you go out for some retail therapy. Make a list of the labels that you feel best in. Look at the colours you wear most often and add to your successful items more of the same.

These clothes will become your uniform. It becomes brainless and painless. Take out the indecision every morning and save time. Be confident.

Get a friend round for an honest opinion. Try on your favourite clothes. Listen to what they say. Have another look and see what they mean. Take on board their suggestions. Let go of the past. Leave room for the future.

The occasion

Think about the different people that you need to be. We all have different personas for different areas of our lives. Get the balance right. Look at your wardrobe. Are you spending enough time at play? Fill in the gaps. Know what you need. Are we what we wear? Take some time to think about it.

The basics

We all need to have a certain amount of clothing basics. These should be in neutral shades, such as black, white or natural, so that they can be mixed and matched to create a wider variety of looks. It also means you don't have to launder as often. It saves time.

Underwear

Have enough for two weeks. Find your favourites – the things that always feel comfortable – and stock up.

Socks/tights

Enough for seven days. If you work out, have the same amount of gym socks. Buy all the same kind to save time in sorting. Keep them in pairs.

T-shirts of neutral colours – black, white, natural or navy x 4

Buy 100 per cent cotton as this allows your skin to breathe. Make sure that they fit really well. Be creative. Dress them up under a suit for casual chic or down for pure relaxation.

Smart shirts/blouses x 5

Mix and match colours and textures. As an alternative to shirts, try silk or rayon bodies or lightweight jumpers in wool, cotton or cashmere.

Relaxed shirts x 5

Try linen. Forget about the wrinkles. Be less confined by going a bit bigger. Feel the fabric. Go for colour.

Smart trousers or skirts x 5

Give yourself choices – black, navy and neutral in solid colours and patterns.

Jackets x 3

Invest in well-cut jackets. Make sure the shoulders fit. Move around when trying them on. Check out the back.

Jumpers x 3

Use them for warmth or instead of a jacket. Choose wool or heavyweight cotton in the winter and lightweight cotton or silk in the summer.

Smart shoes x 4 pairs

Rotate them often. Two pairs should be black. Keep them clean and resole them as soon as they need it.

Casual shoes x 2 pairs

Make them fun and comfortable. Kick around. Hang out.

2 items of outerwear

Think casual. Think smart.

accessorise

Transform the simplest outfit into a sophisticated look in less than a minute. Don't be boring. Go for colour. Add style. Play dress up. Have some options. Maximise the looks you can achieve. My favourites have stood the test of time. Next time you want to buy a new top, buy an accessory instead. Start a collection. Get your act together.

Belts x 3
One black belt, one brown belt and one thin belt. Belts finish the look of an outfit and can be worn over lightweight jumpers to create a 'nipped-in' waist.

Black high heels
Classic cut with great lines. Oh, what they can do to a simple black dress.

Chunky silver necklace
A great way to smarten up a pair of trousers and jumper.

Pearls
Call me old-fashioned, but they worked for Grace Kelly and Audrey Hepburn.

Watches x 2
A funky inexpensive one to hang around in and a more grown-up style for evenings.

Small, black evening bag
Every girl must have one.

Handbags x 2
One big. One small. At least one black. The big one should be able to hold everything you might ever want to carry and can be a substitute for a briefcase or gym bag.

Pashmina shawl
Buy a large shawl in a neutral colour that will go with most of your things. Wear on one shoulder over a blouse to soften the look of a long skirt or trousers, at your neck for warmth, around your shoulders for an evening out or over your legs when travelling. They are lightweight and truly versatile.

Hair accessories
Slides, combs, headbands, chopsticks – whatever suits your hairstyle. Try them out when you are having a bad hair day or when you just want a change.

Earrings x 2 pairs
Although I own tons, I wear two pairs the most. One black and silver with a small drop, and the other my trusted pearls.

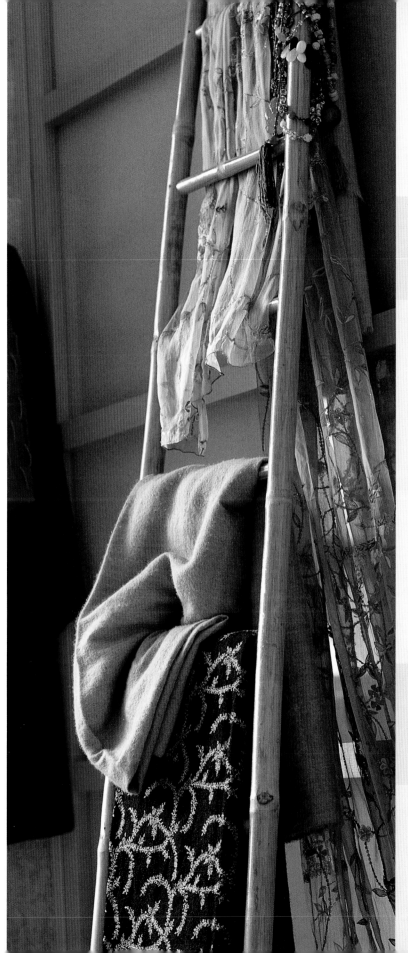

10 things to do before you leave your bedroom

Make your bed.

Hang up any unworn clothes.

Put your shoes away.

Put dirty clothes in the laundry basket.

Bring any dishes or glasses to the kitchen.

Pack your bag for the day.

Throw away any unnecessary papers.

Empty the waste bin.

Turn off the radio.

Turn off the lights.

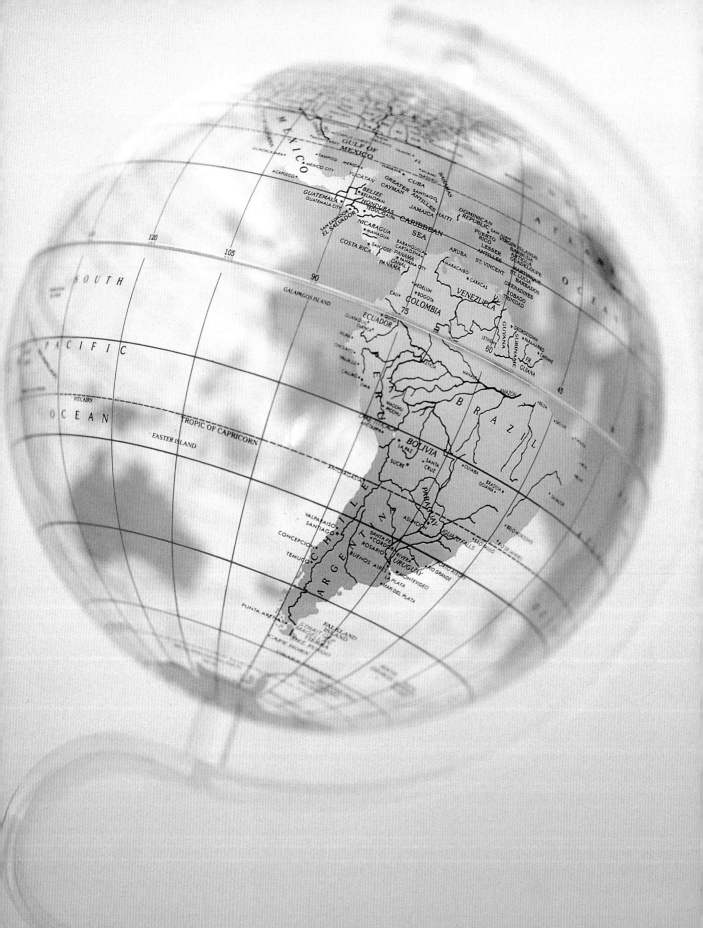

getting around

We spend 20 per cent of our day getting from place to place, which is an astounding amount of time. When you travel every day, delays and other problems are a fact of life. This is not a great way to spend time.

So what are the choices? We have to go to work, transport the kids or go shopping. Start with the right attitude. Never rush. Give yourself time. Drive more slowly. Be thoughtful. Let a car in before you. Don't make it a race. It will change your outlook dramatically. Try it tomorrow.

Save time by being prepared. Get your tickets or change out before you get in the queue. Keep a schedule of transportation times so you know your options. Be flexible. Leave the house five minutes earlier or five minutes later. See what happens. It may save you time.

Be constructive with your time in transit. Read something uplifting or listen to your favourite calming music; catch up with your correspondence; read the newspapers or prepare for your day.

Make eye contact. Say hello to someone you see every day on the bus or train. You may learn something new or make a new friend. Most of all, make it a point not to let the pressures of getting where you need to be ruin your day.

Get out of town. Plan a break. Go somewhere you have never been and take advantage of planning ahead. Save money by booking in advance. Have something to look forward to. Check out the weather. Learn about the culture.

Travel light. Be decisive. Know how to pack. Be prepared to get away at a moment's notice by keeping the essentials packed. When opportunity knocks, be ready, willing and able.

Be resourceful. Getting what you need no longer means leaving your house. Enter the twenty-first century. Discover how to use the Internet and shop on-line or by mail order. Life will never be the same. Knowledge is power. Explore the resources of the world at the touch of a button. Take your time. Don't be impatient. Get connected. Learn to search for the answers. Practice makes perfect. Try until you get it right.

A fifth of every day is too long to be doing something that you don't enjoy. Find a way to make it work for you.

trauma-free travel tips

Feeling like a trapped sardine isn't the best way to start your day. For those of us who seem to spend most of our lives on public transport, it's an all too familiar feeling. There is something very de-humanising about crowded transportation, especially the underground. Take control and explore the options. A few days' worth of research could make a dramatic impact on how you start and end your day. Be creative. Think about the elements of your journey that you most dislike and find ways around them. You could save time and money while improving the quality of your life!

Traveller's etiquette

Regardless of your mode of transport, always be polite. Don't start the day fighting to get on a very crowded train or bus. Wait for the next one. Pay attention to the people around you. If there are passengers that need your seat more than you, offer it to them.

Refrain from eating: hundreds of food odours in a confined space can be unpleasant. Respect people's space. Don't have your music blaring or lots of bags for people to trip over. Make it a pleasant journey for everyone.

Timing is everything

If you travel at peak times (usually around 7.45–9.30am and 4.30–7pm), you are going to find crowds. It's as simple as that. But there are a number of ways to avoid these times.

Experiment over a week by leaving your house at different times. Starting your journey an hour earlier may give you time after you reach your destination for relaxation or exercise. Have a cup of coffee and read the paper. Take your trainers and have a walk around a park. Window shop. Sit on a bench and read a book. Clear the cobwebs from your head before you start your day. You may have a flexible job that would enable you to come in a bit later and stay longer. You never know until you ask.

Be a map reader

Buy a good map that shows all the transportation routes to your destination. It could be one of the best purchases you ever make. Find out all the options of how you can get from A to B. If you hate the underground, look into the bus and train routes as an alternative. Being in the know will get you there with less stress.

The best deal

Research the costs of your commute. Buying weekly or monthly tickets will save you money and time. It will also enable you to travel for socialising without additional expense. Yearly travel passes are the most cost-effective way to use public transport. Check with your employer to see if they would be willing to purchase a yearly ticket and deduct it from your salary.

Car pooling

Investigate the possibility of driving with others going to the same or nearby destinations. You may find that the shared cost of four travelling by car is less than public transport and if you have to use a car, it is more environmentally friendly to share. Chat with people waiting for the train or colleagues who live close to you. Explore all the options to make your journey as pleasant as possible.

Get fit

Walking or bicycling to work can dramatically improve your physical condition and mental outlook on life. It can also save you lots of money. An hour's brisk walk or bike ride will improve your cardiovascular system and tone up your muscles. Keep alert and pay attention to the things around you – you'll see things that you pass every day in a totally new light. Remember always to wear the proper gear and pay attention to the rules of the road if you're cycling in the city.

Viva Italia

When in Rome (or even when you're not), do as the Romans and drive a scooter. In urban areas the world over scooters are becoming one of the primary means of transportation. Gas-efficient and easy to park, they are a quick way of getting around. Always wear a helmet and drive with care.

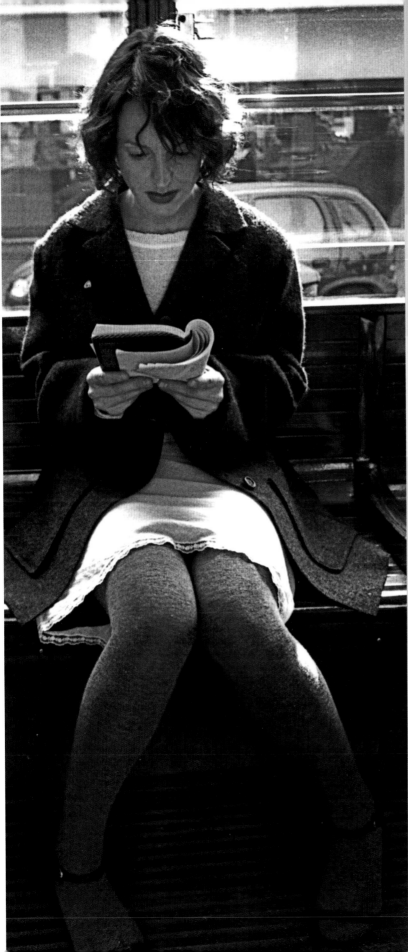

10 things to do on public transport

Always be prepared and have your tickets ready when you need them.

Sort out your loose change for your ticket, coffee or a paper.

Read the paper or your favourite spiritual book.

Listen to your favourite music – softly.

Keep a journal.

Review your papers for the day.

Write a letter.

Plan a party.

Smile at a stranger.

Pay attention to things around you.

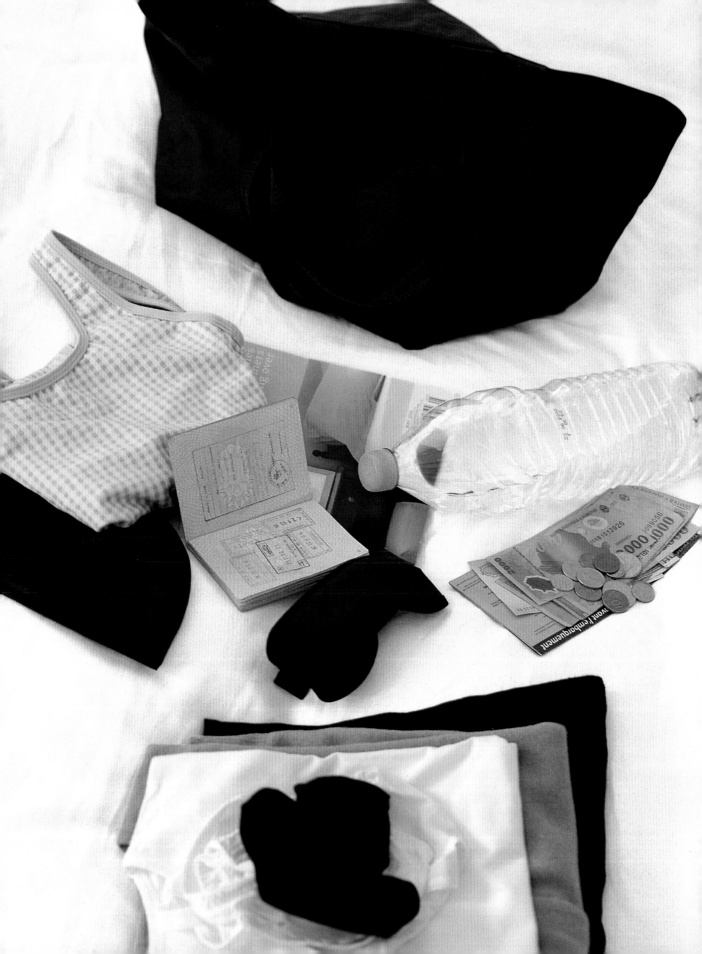

planning a trip

Be it for business or pleasure, a trip anywhere can be either a great adventure, if you're relaxed and in control, or a big bore, if the process of getting there is a nightmare!

I love to travel. Anywhere, any time. The thought of an adventure fills me with joy and excitement. I like to plan a trip well in advance so that I can look forward to it and use it as a motivator to keep me going, especially when planning a winter holiday.

I have lost luggage, missed one plane and suffered countless delays. I've had awful hotel rooms and amazing hotel rooms, fabulous weather and miserable weather that I was totally unprepared for. Most importantly, I have learned a lot about travelling.

Follow the famous Boy Scout motto and Be Prepared – not necessarily for everything but for most things. Frequent business travellers might need to hop on a plane at a few hours' notice. For a family with kids, husbands included, getting to a destination without all your possessions can end in tears.

Do a bit of research. Check out the likely weather forecast and find out what you will be doing when you get there. This is essential in planning your wardrobe and all those other things that life can be miserable without.

Always keep a fully stocked essentials kit ready and waiting. No matter how infrequently you travel, having the essentials prepared gives you one less thing to have to organise. The basics should be: toothbrush, toothpaste, razor, medication, plasters, eye-care products and all those essential toiletries that you can't live without.

To make your temporary home feel more like your own home, take a few special things as well: your favourite perfume, a scented candle and a small photo to put by your bed. Don't forget an alarm clock if time will be of the essence. Customise your kit to reflect your purpose for travelling by adding any seasonal or regional necessities.

Essential kits for children should contain all the things that will keep them entertained throughout the journey. This is the one time when more is better than less. What is their favourite toy of the moment? Bring it.

Before you start to pack, decide which cases or bags you will be taking. I am almost as bad with luggage as I am with shoes – many for each occasion. I personally prefer soft luggage with millions of pockets. This helps me when I am travelling to lots of destinations on one trip as everything always goes in the same place and I know when I have left something behind. It is all about personal choice. Carry a small bag with you for the things you can't live without. Always tag your luggage on both the inside and the outside with contact phone numbers of your destination.

10 things to carry in your hand luggage

Essentials kit.

Passport, tickets, money.

Book or something to keep you amused.

Eyeshades, headrest, earplugs.

One change of underwear.

Bathing suit (or hat and gloves if more appropriate).

Socks.

One change of clothes.

Shawl, wrap or jumper.

Big bottle of water.

packing a suitcase

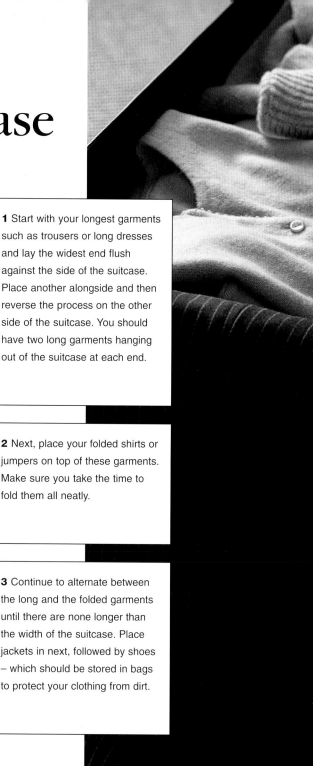

Always remember that somewhere during your trip you will have to carry your luggage on your own. No matter how many valets or luggage carts you have, somewhere that luggage will be yours to carry. This should make you think seriously about how much you pack.

The first thing to consider is the look you want to have when you get there – professional, casual chic or a combination? Create a mix and match uniform that enables you to make fewer items go further. Stick with a basic colour scheme like black or white and add a few accent colours to change the look. Don't forget accessories: they can dramatically alter any outfit and transform daytime into evening. They also require very little packing space. Think about your top 10 accessories that you would like to take with you, from belts to earrings.

If you are able, give yourself time to think about your packing. Lay out all the clothes you would like to take for a day or two. Then edit them down to the things that you really think you should take. You know what they say – less is more. Edit again.

When you have selected your clothes, you can begin to pack. Packing a suitcase is like making a lasagne – good layering is essential. Follow these steps for an easy way to avoid wrinkles and, hence, unnecessary ironing when you finally arrive at your destination.

1 Start with your longest garments such as trousers or long dresses and lay the widest end flush against the side of the suitcase. Place another alongside and then reverse the process on the other side of the suitcase. You should have two long garments hanging out of the suitcase at each end.

2 Next, place your folded shirts or jumpers on top of these garments. Make sure you take the time to fold them all neatly.

3 Continue to alternate between the long and the folded garments until there are none longer than the width of the suitcase. Place jackets in next, followed by shoes – which should be stored in bags to protect your clothing from dirt.

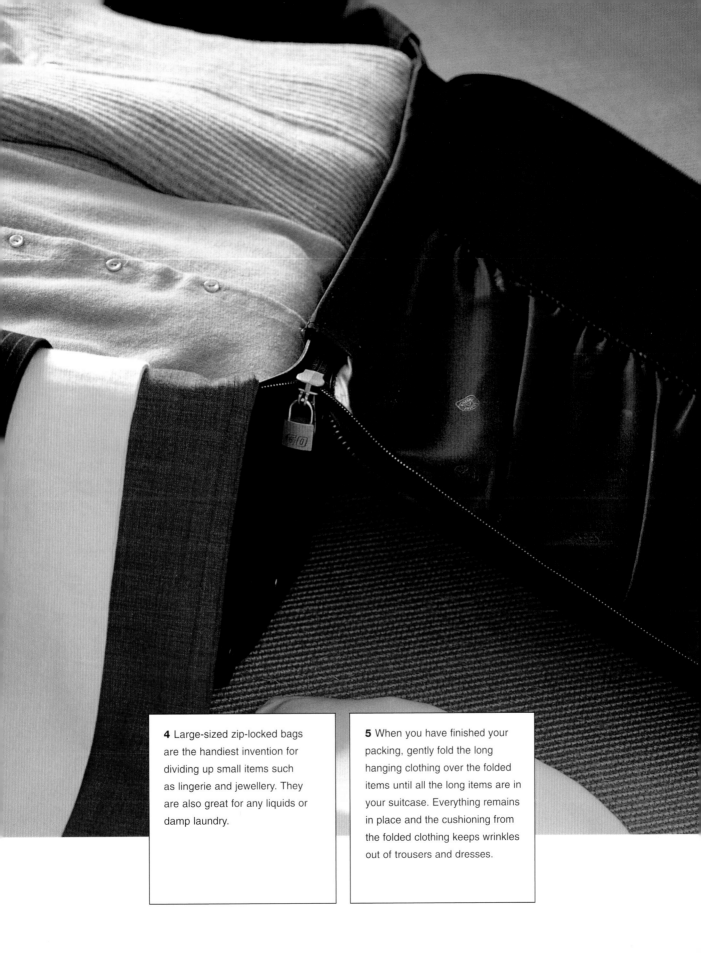

4 Large-sized zip-locked bags are the handiest invention for dividing up small items such as lingerie and jewellery. They are also great for any liquids or damp laundry.

5 When you have finished your packing, gently fold the long hanging clothing over the folded items until all the long items are in your suitcase. Everything remains in place and the cushioning from the folded clothing keeps wrinkles out of trousers and dresses.

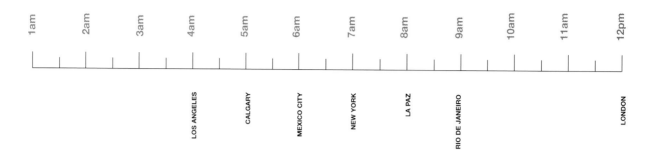

jet lag

Air travel means that exotic foreign destinations are now only hours away, but there is a downside to travelling vast distances in a short time – the dreaded jet lag.

Jet lag can make you feel like you are on a strange planet – almost like being in the Twilight Zone. The reality is that you are a time traveller, racing through time zones and throwing your body clock out of whack. The earth rotates on its axis once every 24 hours and the electromagnetic system of your body, your biological clock, is controlled by this 24-hour cycle. You need to wind it up and reset it to get with the flow.

It is said that it can take one day to recuperate from each time zone change you make. Who wants to be out of it for that long? Most people suffer more heading east, as reflected in the saying, 'East's a beast and west is best.' However, there are things you can do to reduce your tiredness when travelling and get back on your feet.

Alternative jet lag cures

1 Trace the inner sole of your shoes onto brown paper with the shiny side down – trust me, there is a shiny side. Place the paper soles inside your shoes. I am told that a top Hollywood executive swears by this! So does my well-travelled friend Kate.

2 Free Press travel writer Gerry Volgenau recommends shining a bright light on the back of both your knees for a short time before you fly. There is no scientific proof that this really helps with jet lag, but the theory is that shining a bright light on this thin-skinned area will affect the natural secretion of melatonin within your body, a hormone that tells you when you are in need of sleep.

3 Eliminating fatty foods from your diet for 48 hours prior to travel can also help. Eat plenty of carbohydrates and vegetables during your flight and, whenever possible, choose the healthy option or vegetarian choice on the airline menu. Some of these may require pre-booking with the airline, so don't forget. Even if it doesn't help to eliminate jet lag, it's great for your waistline.

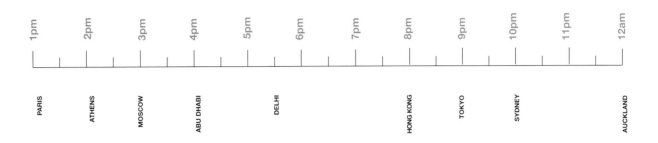

1pm 2pm 3pm 4pm 5pm 6pm 7pm 8pm 9pm 10pm 11pm 12am

PARIS ATHENS MOSCOW ABU DHABI DELHI HONG KONG TOKYO SYDNEY AUCKLAND

top 10 time traveller tips

Always wear comfortable clothing to travel. This doesn't mean that you have to look scruffy, just think about wearing loose-fitting clothes so that you feel less restricted.

Change your watch to the local time of your destination as soon as you get on the plane. Pretend you are there already and live by their time, sleeping and eating at the appropriate times.

Drink 225–350ml (8–12fl oz) of mineral water every hour. You may think you'll get sick of drinking, but it does work in helping you to avoid dehydration. It is also very good for you.

Take care of your skin. Apply lotion liberally before boarding the plane and frequently during the flight, particularly on face and hands. Spray mineral water on your face for an instant pick-me-up. Bring essential oils to inhale.

Be sure to move around. Many airlines now show videos of in-flight exercises for passengers. Take a walk and stretch your back and limbs every few hours.

Limit your alcohol consumption. I know it sounds very boring, especially on long-haul flights at the start of your holiday, but it can dehydrate you and tire you.

Always carry eye shades, a pillow and earplugs in your hand luggage, as they are the best way to tune out the cabin activity when it's time to sleep. The pillow can also give your neck support when you are sitting for prolonged periods.

When you arrive at your destination, ground yourself to rebalance the electromagnetic charge in your body. Try walking barefoot on the ground or swimming in the ocean for at least 15–20 minutes. You will be shocked at the difference it can make.

Stand in direct sunlight for 10–20 minutes without sunglasses, being careful to avoid eye damage by not looking directly into the sun. This helps to orient your body clock to the proper time zone. Remember, though, to apply sun cream with a high sun protection factor (SPF) to avoid any damage to your skin.

Acclimatise yourself to the local time zone by taking meals at the proper time. Try not to nap during the day, as it will be more difficult to get into a normal sleep pattern, unless of course you always take a siesta. Stay up until at least 10pm and try to get at least six hours' sleep every night.

on the road

Travelling by car can be a real adventure – beautiful scenery, lovely roads, getting away – but it can also be the trip from hell. Be prepared and stay amused is my motto for getting my kicks on Route 66.

Be prepared

The inside of your car is where you're going to be, so clean it. Make sure all the layers of dust are removed from both inside and outside the windows to give you a clean outlook. Give the whole car a thorough vacuum and throw away all the rubbish under your seats and in the glove compartment. Wipe down the instrument panel and make sure that you can read the speedometer – you don't want be caught out going way too fast.

Check all the essentials: oil, fuel, tyre pressure, windscreen fluid. Make sure that you have a spare tyre, a spanner, a jack and some water for emergencies. Bring a spare set of car keys that you carry with you at all times – just in case. Keep any vehicle or insurance documents locked in your glove compartment, along with any roadside assistance cards. Spare change at your fingertips is a must for any road tolls or quick phone-box stops. Keep an emergency first aid kit and an old blanket in the car: you never know when you might need them.

Know where you are going. Get out the maps and mark the pages. If there is a designated map-reader, make sure they do their homework and study the route before you begin. Tempers can flare when you've missed the turning for the third time. Remember to bring your reading glasses if you need them – they will be essential!

Stay amused

Keep the creature comforts close to hand. Ideally, your car will be equipped with a holder for your cappuccino and have a great stereo – two things that can make the trip seem like a holiday. Plan your tunes well; choose a variety of all your favourites to cover every mood, particularly if your journey is long.

Kids and pets need to be amused too. Children are easily bored and you do not want the holiday to start off with frustration or tears. Personal headsets, Gameboys or favourite toys can distract the kids for part of the time, but if you can, also play some car games as a group. Find the alphabet in order on number plates or play I-Spy – the old ones are often the best.

If you have pets, they need to see out of the window and have a good sniff of what's going on outside the car. Cover the seats with an old blanket and bring along some chews and water. Never bring a squeaky toy – it will drive you to distraction. To let them drink without mess, keep a plastic bowl in the car that you can fill during the journey.

All but the kitchen sink

When packing, keep anything you might need during your journey or for an overnight stop in the boot, but If there's no room for people when you've finished packing the car, stop in the name of love. If you're not comfortable the chances are the trip will be doomed from the start. You need to go back to the packing basics. Make sure you've been decisive and limited yourself to the bare essentials. If there is still no room in the car, there's no way but up: it's the roof or nowhere.

Start with a good, solid roof-rack that you firmly attach to the car. Remember the laws of aerodynamics and make sure to minimise any wind resistance by always stacking luggage horizontally and distributing the weight evenly across the whole roof.

Put your heaviest suitcases on the bottom layer and keep stacking according to the weight of the luggage. When complete, cover the luggage pile on the roof-rack with a waterproof tarpaulin and secure it down at the corners and sides with bungee cords.

When driving, try not to make any sudden stops or you could find all your luggage crashing around your ears. And take care when driving around corners so that the weight of the luggage doesn't unbalance the car. If you're properly prepared, you'll get to your destination with no trouble at all and will have had some fun on the way.

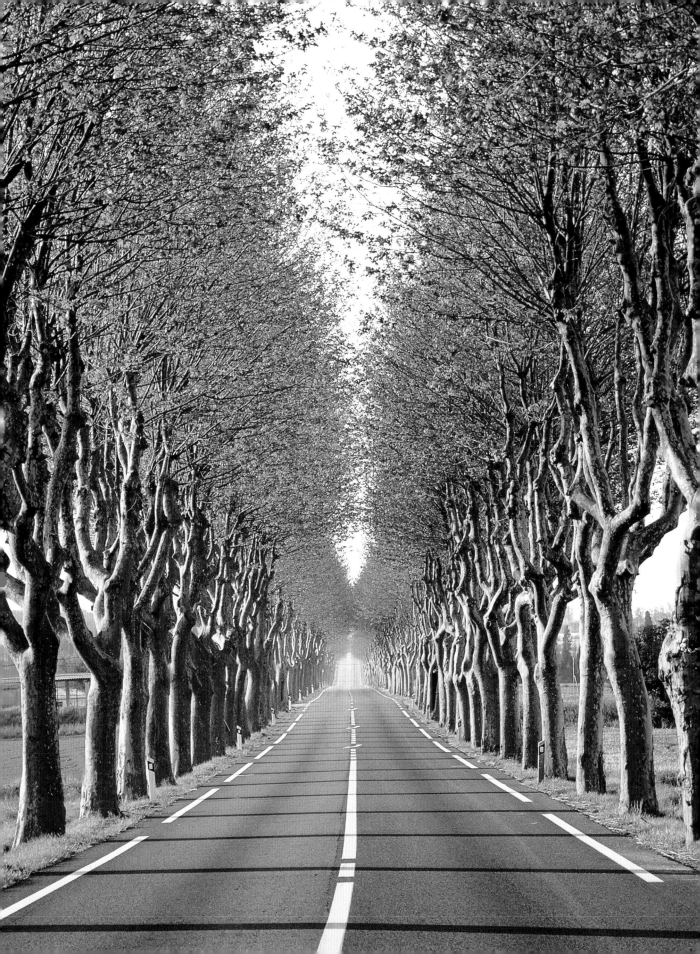

navigating the superhighway

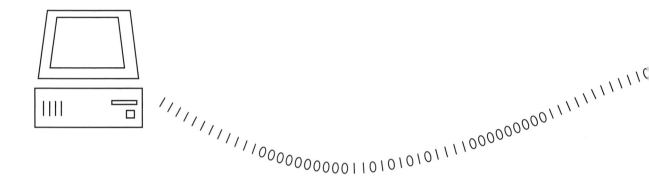

If getting around is getting you down, try finding a way to get what you need from the comfort of your own home.

Our homes have become far more than a place to hang our hat at the end of the day. Each year, more and more of us work from home. Over 30 per cent of the population in America and the United Kingdom own computers. We are now able to communicate with anyone around the world at the touch of a button and the cost of a local phone call. We are even able to access the Internet from our television set. And the next 10 years could bring even more technology to our fingertips.

All kids are computer literate; most know more than their parents. If you know where to look, the Internet can save you time. You can find the answer to any question. You can book travel, buy anything from anywhere in the world, visit public art galleries, get news and chat with friends without leaving your home. Don't let fear stop you from

getting switched on. You have to start somewhere and there is no time like the present. All you need is a computer, a modem, a telephone line (a dedicated line makes life easier) and access to the Internet via a service provider.

Basic lingo

There are a number of terms that you will come across as you find out more about computers. If you know these terms it is much easier to understand exactly what your own requirements are.

Modem

Either internally built into your computer or externally connected, this translates your computer's output to digital so that data can be sent through the telecommunications network both to and from your computer.

Internet

International network of computers that are linked to exchange information.

Service Provider

Networked computers that provide access to the Internet. You are probably bombarded with special offers daily. Check around for the best option for you. The catch is always the cost of phone time. Read the small print and ask questions.

Email

Electronic mail allows you to get an electronic letter instantly to anyone in the world with an email address. You will be given an address and access by your service provider.

WWW

World Wide Web is the way in which we navigate the data on the Internet.

Search Engine

Think of this as the card file in your library. You type in what you are looking for and it gives you a listing of web pages that relate to your query.

Who is dot com, anyway?

Every service, company or person on the Internet has a registered name or address. If the address has .com at the end of it this indicates that the service is a company. Many countries such as the United Kingdom use their country code at the end of their web address, as in www.theholdingcompany.co.uk, to indicate that it is a UK company. United States addresses most often end with .com. Non-commercial institutions have different endings. Educational facilities end in .edu; government sites end in .gov; and non-profit organisations end in .org. Knowing the endings will help you figure out an address. Start with www., add the company name, usually in lower-case letters without any spaces, and end with the appropriate suffix. Each country has a different code: for example, Australia (au); Canada (ca); France (fr); Germany (de); Hong Kong (hk); Indonesia (id); Japan (jp) and Netherlands (nl).

Getting connected

Once you have decided on a service provider, you will usually receive a CD-ROM or disk that will take you through the installation process. All service providers are geared up for offering help to novices, so if you can't figure it out, get on.the phone. Better yet, find a computer literate mate to take you through it.

Your service provider will provide you with a web browser (the most popular are Microsoft Internet Explorer and Netscape Communicator). These are software programs that let you do just that – browse the web, or 'surf' as it is sometimes known. As you spend more time on the Internet you will learn how to do things more quickly.

You will also be issued with lots of personal details – including user name, passwords and an email address. Write them down somewhere safe. If you are anything like me you will forget them. If you have a choice, pick a user name

and password that you are likely to remember. You will sometimes be issued with a hint to remind you, such as 'black poodle' to indicate that you have used your dog's name as a password.

You are now ready to start. Connect your modem to the telephone line. Click on the icon for your dial-up connection and away you go. With some service providers you may have to type in your password and user name at this point before a connection is attempted; with my service provider I have to type in my password and user name once an initial connection has been made. There may be a box on the screen that says 'remember password'. Click it and the computer will remember this for you so you don't have to. While a connection is being sought your modem will make a loud, continuous buzzing / screeching / popping sound, so don't be alarmed. Once you're connected the world is at your fingertips.

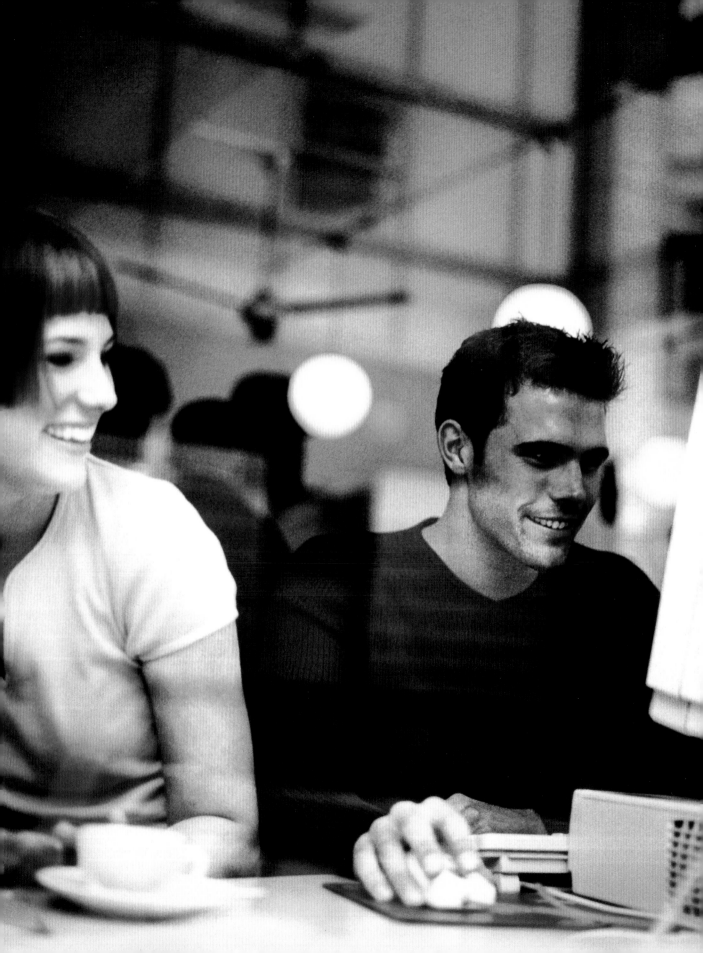

Patience is a virtue

If it didn't work, don't give up. The essential thing is to get the set-up right. Sometimes it's as easy as plugging your modem into your telephone line or making sure you have the correct phone number. If you've checked everything and it still doesn't work, give it one more go and write down what is happening, paying attention to sounds and error messages.

Call your provider. They really will hold your hand and talk you through it step by step. If you are continuously hear the engaged tone continuously, you and the entire universe may be trying to get on-line. Try again at an off-peak time. If it still doesn't work, you may want to change providers.

Everybody's gone surfing

You have arrived. You are connected and have power in those fingertips to access any information or service you require. You will automatically be connected to the home page of your provider, which is the springboard for exploring the web. There will be tons of advertising to lure you away from your mission. Stay focused. There are two ways of accessing web sites. The first is to type in the address at the top of your screen where it says 'address' or 'go to'. There is no need to type http//:. Type in the address starting with www., press the return key on the keyboard and away you go. The second way is to click on a link. Whenever you see an address in the information that you are searching for, clicking on the address will link you to the site. To return to your home page, click your heels three times

(just like Dorothy in The Wizard of Oz) and press the home button on the top of your screen and you will be back on familiar territory.

Seek and you can find

The fastest way to get information is by using a search engine or search directory. These are huge databases that constantly search the millions of web pages and store information. Know how to search. When you type in the name of the item you wish to find, be as specific as possible to limit the amount of irrelevant information you may retrieve.

Each word in the search is treated individually unless you tell the search that all the words you have asked for must be found together. To do so, use quotation marks to enclose the phrase. Typing Jet Lag Remedies would bring up lots of information on jets or remedies, or even lagging, but not necessarily what you are looking for. Typing "Jet Lag Remedies" with the quotation marks around it requires the search engine to look for all the words together. It's as simple as that.

Every day, thousands of new sites go on-line. Many won't be around for long. A search engine should be able to locate the up-to-date information. My favourite search directory is www.google.com. It has a no-nonsense user-friendly screen without the hype of advertising. Don't get fooled into searching retail sites for general information, as they are just trying to sell you something. Try searching these 10 selected sites for the same thing and see which works best for you.

10 search engines and directories

Alta Vista
www.av.com

Britannica
www.britannica.com

Google
www.google.com

Goto
www.goto.com

Excite
www.excite.com

HotBot
www.hotbot.com

InfoSeek
www.infoseek.com

Lycos
www.lycos.com

Northern Light
www.nlsearch.com

Yahoo
www.yahoo.com

10 quick retail therapy fixes

Auctions – www.ebay.com

Books, CDs, Videos –
www.amazon.co.uk
www.amazon.com (USA)

Cosmetics – www.origins.com
www.clinique.com

Flowers – www.interflora.com

Home – www.conran.co.uk
www.theholdingcompany.co.uk

Pet Products –
www.petsmart.com (USA)
www.petspyjamas.co.uk

Travel – www.lastminute.com
www.lastminutetravel.com (USA)

home shopping

The biggest shop in the world

If you don't want the hassle of the high street, shopping from home makes sense. Although you will have access to shops around the world, they don't all mail abroad. Check their policy as soon as you log-on in order to avoid disappointment.

Despite many rumours to the contrary, your card details can be more protected on-line than when you go into a high-street shop. Most retail sites use secure servers, which means that no one has access except you and them. I shop on-line all the time and have never encountered any problems.

You can compare prices on-line and get some great bargains in the process. Most on-line retailers will mail the goods immediately and will let you know by email when to expect your package. Check the small print for return policies and any shipping charges that may apply, just in case.

Most major chains of supermarkets now provide an on-line shopping service with delivery straight to your kitchen. A small surcharge is worth the time you save. Call your local store for details. Don't get frustrated by your initial order, as it can take hours to search through the aisles and put together a shopping list. Your initial order is then stored in the memory – just add any new items for further orders. Remember to order several days before you need the goods.

Mail-order magic

Like on-line retailers, mail-order companies can deliver things right to your door without you ever needing to face the crowds. If you want to buy clothing, it is best if you are already familiar with the brand and, therefore, the likely quality and fit of the clothing. Pictures can be deceiving and something that may look enormous in a photo can actually turn out to be much smaller than anticipated. Make sure you ask the dimensions if you are ordering anything that needs to fit in a specific location. Repackaging and posting returns can be time-consuming and sometimes costly.

A few mail-order companies only take the initial orders from the public and are not involved with delivery. If this is the case the items you purchase are likely to come directly from the manufacturer. This means that if you order a number of items you could end up receiving them all individually. You not only need to keep track of how much of your order has been supplied, but also may have to be at home to sign for the parcels. If you think the mail-order company you have used may work in this way, double-check where your parcels are coming from and when they should be arriving so that no misunderstandings arise.

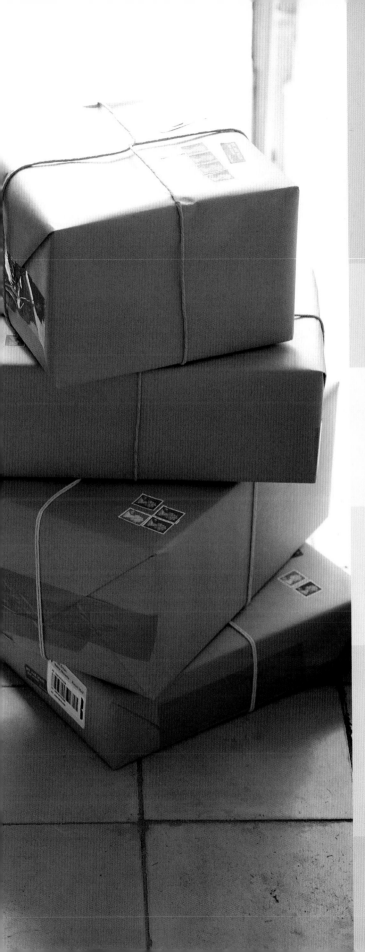

10 great reasons to shop by post

Some great mail-order companies do not have retail outlets.

You can find more specialised products.

You usually get more information from a catalogue than from a shop assistant.

You can order things from around the world.

I can avoid looking at myself in badly lit full-length mirrors in shop dressing rooms.

I can order my favourite things that I know fit over and over again.

It's the perfect way to send a gift. Most will wrap your gift and send a handwritten note with your message. I'd do anything to avoid going to the Post Office.

Every time a parcel arrives for me it seems like a present.

Sometimes you have to live with things before you know they are going to work. Having a mail-order catalogue at home, you can check it out before you make the mistake.

It saves lots and lots of time.

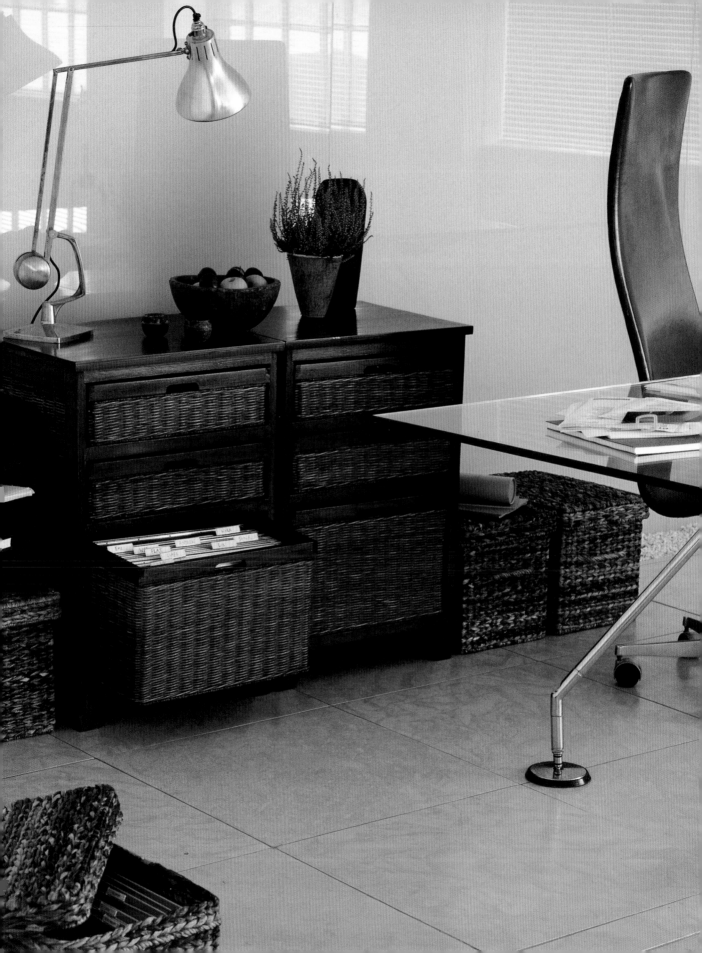

nine to five

"Whatever you can do or dream you can, begin it. Boldness has genius, magic and power in it. Begin it now." GOETHE

You are extremely fortunate if you are passionate about what you do to earn a living: to wake up every day and be inspired; to put your heart and soul into everything you create; to feel fulfilled.

There can be nothing worse than dreading every day because the thought of going to work is so unpleasant. Life is too short. Getting a life means getting to grips with the situation and doing what only you know you are truly meant to do.

Try to learn something new every day and remember it. Focus on what is going on around you. Communicate with all the people that you work with. Don't take anything for granted.

Your workplace, be it home or away, needs to be stimulating. You need to be able to share ideas and learn new tricks. You need to be able to communicate.

Most of my best ideas are born from talking things through with co-workers or friends. Creativity inspires creativity. It's a great buzz when people are on the same wavelength. I'm sure you have all experienced how positive group energy can feel. With a little bit of inspiration, you can conquer the world.

Sit down and make a list of what you love about your work. Then think about what really frustrates you. Take control of your life and think about how to change the things you don't like and then take the first step. Make it happen.

If your job requires you to come into contact with the public, really listen to what they say. You will learn something. Put yourself in their shoes and think about how you would act if you were in their situation. Whenever someone

makes a complaint to me I always ask them what they would do if they were me. The answers are very interesting.

Working from home requires a huge amount of self-discipline due to the many distractions and lack of social interaction. Try to set aside a space that you can call your office and develop a daily schedule. Make sure that you have all the necessary information for the project on which you are working. Get the job done and appreciate that it's a great luxury to be in the comfort of your own home.

Remember: we're here for a good time, not a long time. Make sure that you have no regrets about not fulfilling your life's ambition; or make sure that you are fulfilling it. If you have a dream, just do it. What have you really got to lose?

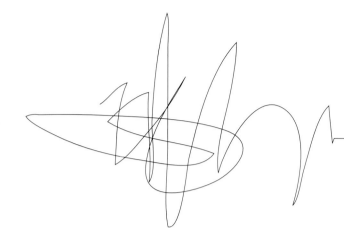

all wound up

Stress is the tension caused by not being in control of a situation. Control means that you have all the right physical and emotional tools needed to achieve the desired result in a given situation. It doesn't mean that you have to control every situation, because that itself can cause stress to both yourself and those around you.

There are many causes of stress – physical, emotional and behavioural – but the feelings of anxiety remain the same. They can manifest themselves physically, with unexplained illnesses and ailments, or emotionally, with symptoms of bad concentration, low energy and a general feeling of being 'down'. The only way to alleviate stress is to take a long look at the cause and make any necessary changes in your job, situation or lifestyle. Life is too short for you to be unhappy.

I believe that deep down inside we all know the truth about any situation. We may not wish to confront the truth, but until we do, it will always be lurking in the background waiting to come out. Always listen to your inner voice if you want to know the way forward.

Environmental cause

You may not think that your environment can make you feel stressed, but sometimes it's as simple as that. We are all affected differently by light, colour, sounds, smells and the space around us. Any one of these factors can contribute to our feelings of being on edge. If we are not comfortable in our space, it is unlikely that we will be successful in achieving our goals. Our inability to accomplish what we set out to do leads to feelings of inadequacy, which inevitably leads to stress.

We can usually cope with physical conditions quite easily. Take a good look around your work space and see how it feels. Do the colours stimulate you or make you feel depressed? Ask if you can change the colour of the walls and go for something that will enhance your level of vitality and creativity. If painting the walls is not possible, use colourful accessories in your office. Bring in some art to hang on the wall or put flowers on your desk. Bright cushions on your chair can also add a bit of life to a depressing space and make the tension disappear.

Sunlight and artificial lights can also have a dramatic impact on our feelings of wellbeing. If you have the chance to switch offices to one with more natural light, go for it. If that is not possible, go out and get a great lamp with warm tones to focus your attention on the work at hand. There are bulbs that offer a more natural light – try to find one of these for the office and use it every day. Good light helps you to accomplish your tasks and will reduce eye strain and headaches.

Tension can also come from being physically uncomfortable. Perhaps you get headaches or have back pain from sitting in a chair that does not give you adequate support. Again, rectify this by asking for a better chair that will support your back and keep you pain-free. If you're feeling great then you can only be more productive.

Make sure that the temperature of your workplace is not causing you to feel ill at ease. Dress according to the usual temperature of the office – remember that in air-conditioned buildings it will remain cool inside even if it is baking outside.

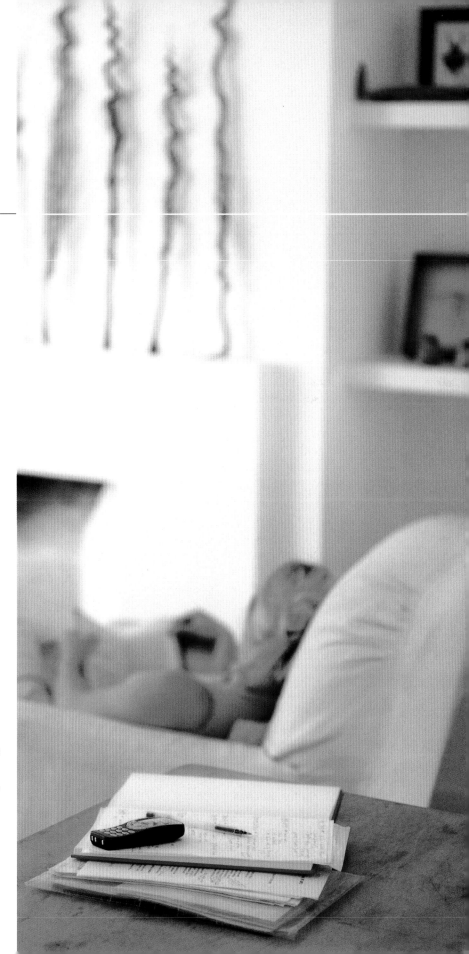

Calm and collected

Deep breathing can calm you in minutes. If the air you breathe is stuffy or smoke-filled it can leave you feeling low on energy. Potted plants will help by adding oxygen to the air.

Essential oils can fill the room with therapeutic benefits to alleviate stress and improve concentration. Try basil or lemon to focus the mind, bergamot for calm and ylang-ylang to reduce anger. You may also feel claustrophobic if you spend too much in confined spaces. Practise your breathing often or leave the office for 20 minutes to gain a different perspective.

Once you've addressed the physical and emotional problems, you have taken the first step towards reducing tension and being happy in your workplace. If you really feel the problems are physical and can't be sorted, at least you have realised what you need in a work environment to enjoy your job and be happy. If they are not achievable in your current job, perhaps it's time to start searching for a new job in a space that is more conducive to your wellbeing.

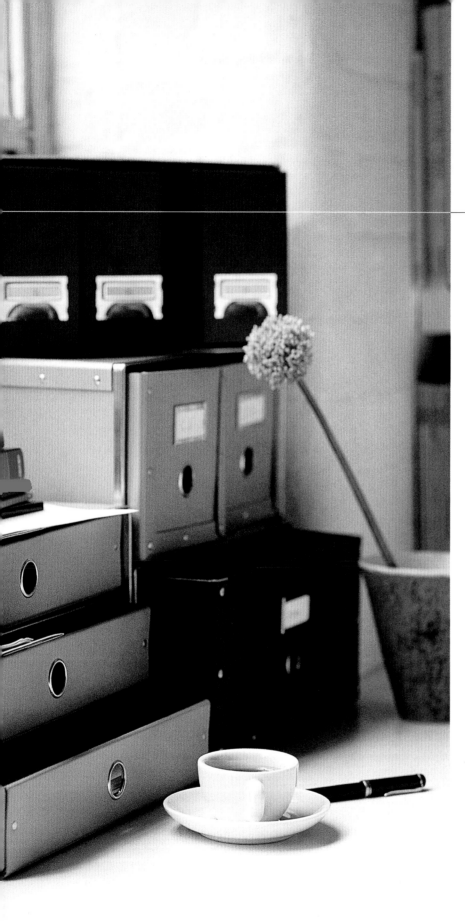

Achieving goals

In order to achieve your goals you first need to decide whether they are all realistic. If you know that you have truly done the best that you can do and you are still unable to achieve your goal, then perhaps you have been unrealistic in your expectations. Give yourself a break. Rome, as we all know, was not built in a day. It was a step-by-step process involving many individuals.

Break down the bigger goals into steps and take it one step at a time. Write them down: they seem more important that way. Never be afraid to ask for help. It is not a sign of weakness. It shows an eagerness to grow and most often can be the first step in making things better. You must always want to make things better!

All the other stuff

In order to feel good about ourselves on the job, most of us need to think that we will accomplish what we set out to do, when we say we'll do it, and that once it's done it will be appreciated by others. We become stressed when any of these are difficult to achieve.

get to grips with your organisational skills

We all suffer from occasional stress brought on by situations. Unrealistic deadlines or our co-workers' bad moods happen in every group situation from time to time. Look back and laugh about it when the situation passes. It is when you feel stressed that, more often than not, you really need to take a few deep breaths and let it go.

A day late and a dollar short

Look at the reasons why you are unable to meet deadlines. Sometimes, in an effort to please others, we say yes when we really mean no. When you agree to do something that you know you can't do, you are creating a no-win situation where everyone will end up disappointed. Tell the truth from the start and eliminate the stress.

If you always think you can get things done and never seem to be able to do it, you must have a searching look at how effectively you work. If you are constantly spending a long time trying to find the things you need to do the job effectively, then you must get to grips with your organisational skills and start from the beginning again.

Go through all your papers and set up an appropriate filing system that will allow you to find everything easily. File all the things you have completed and get rid of anything that you no longer need. A clean desk promotes clear thinking.

You must set daily targets and make sure that you are completing them on most days. This means that you have to take the time to plan your day and dedicate yourself to beginning and finishing projects in order of priority. If you have a tendency to procrastinate, do your least favourite jobs first and leave the most enjoyable for last.

Don't get distracted. Focus on the job at hand and don't move on until it is complete. Persistence always pays off – particularly when you don't like doing something. You will feel a tremendous sense of accomplishment and relief that you are moving forward.

If you really are unable to finish an assignment, stop and think about what it was that prevented you from getting the job done. Deal with it there and then and learn from it. If there are too many phone calls, don't take them.

If co-workers come in and chat, keep your door closed or say that you're sorry but you don't have the time. Knowing how and when to say no is an important step in getting control of your life. Think about it.

Pat on the back

We all have a need to be appreciated in everything we do. My best advice is to let the appreciation come from within. Take the first step and give yourself a big pat on the back when you have done something that you are proud of. Be happy in the knowledge that you have succeeded at accomplishing what you set out to do.

Don't worry about what other people think. You know the truth. You dedicated yourself to getting the job done and you did it. This simple bit of truth can make a difference in all areas of your life. It can and will alleviate stress. Be confident about your abilities and recognise the skills that you have. Think positively and you will accomplish more. Believe that you will succeed and you will. Think calm and you will be calm. Look at how much power you really have and use it.

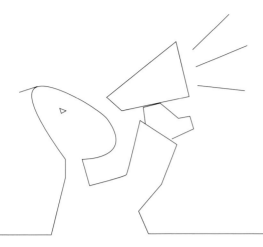

10 tips for effective communication

Remember the game you used to play as a kid when you all sat around in a circle and the first person whispered something to the next person and it went on and on until the last person said what they heard. Inevitably, after the phrase had gone from person to person, the end result always differed dramatically from what was initially said. In a simple child's game, you can learn the rules of communication.

Go straight to the source
Never trust hearsay. Always go directly to the source and you will always get to the bottom of the situation. We all believe things we hear from other people and it always leads to trouble.

Listen to what people say
Concentrate not on your inner thoughts, but on what people say to you. Don't interrupt or finish other people's sentences – it is not a competition. Make sure that you completely understand what the other person is saying. Always ask for clarification and repeat what you think you have heard. Take notes during the conversation to remind yourself of any further action that may need to happen as a result of your conversation.

Put yourself in their shoes
Always try to view a situation from both sides. Think about the circumstances that caused someone to react in a particular manner and then think about what you would do in the same situation. You might find you would have done the same thing. If not, think about why you would have handled it differently and present your case.

Think before you speak
Don't let the emotions of the moment cause you to say something that you can never take back. Words are a powerful tool that can wound unnecessarily. Before you say a single word, give yourself five minutes to plan your argument or point so that it is expressed in the most positive way possible.

You don't have to have the last … word

Make a conscious effort not to always have the last word. Practice makes perfect.

Don't read between the lines

Live in the here and now. If you listened to what you were told and repeated what was said, take it at face value. Do not try to interpret what someone is thinking – you can't get inside their head and it will only lead to misunderstandings.

If possible, do it in person

If you have something difficult to discuss, the best way to do it is face to face. Don't hide behind a computer screen or engage in a war of paper. It always makes matters worse. Take the time to arrange a one-on-one meeting. Look people straight in the eye when you are talking to them. Try to keep emotions out of it and stick to the facts.

Be concise

Whether speaking on the phone or penning a letter, be as brief as you can. Include all the relevant details, what action you wish to be taken and the date you need a result. If the date passes without a response, call or write again. Always keep notes of all the actions you have taken, including the date and time.

Be positive

Whether answering the phone, writing a letter or meeting someone face to face, always be upbeat and positive. It will dramatically change the outcome of any situation. Positive energy can diffuse even the most difficult situations. Give it a go. Always visualise a happy ending and you will see that things work better.

Know when to let go

In the grand scheme of life, some things just aren't that important. Don't harbour grudges. Once you have communicated your thoughts, move on. Happiness, health and peace of mind are all that really matter. Never forget it!

getting on with it

Planning is the only effective way to make sure that you get the job done. There is no way round it. If you don't know where you're going, it's going to take you a very long time to get there. We all need directions to find the way – a daily A–Z.

My mother always told me that there is nothing you can't accomplish if you just set your mind to it and where there is a will there is a way. I believed her. Believe it too and you will succeed in whatever you set out to do.

So every day, first thing in the morning, set your mind to achieving your daily goals. Tell yourself you need a plan of how to accomplish them and then forget about it. Eat your breakfast, walk to work or go to the gym. A perfect example of how this works is a situation we have all been in. You bump into someone that you've met before and can't think of their name. The more you try, the more difficult it becomes. It can be quite embarrassing – particularly if they remember yours! The minute they've gone and you forget about it, the name will pop into your head. It's true, isn't it? You planted the idea that you wanted to know the name and your subconscious delivered. It goes back to the theory that we all know the truth about any situation if we give ourselves the opportunity to listen to it. Start now. Write down the first things that come into your mind and there is your plan. Believe it and it will work for you.

Happy endings

Always visualise a positive ending. It makes a dramatic difference. If you believe you can achieve, you will. List the steps that it will take to achieve the positive outcome and then dedicate 100 per cent of your energy to achieving it. It really is as simple as that. Let nothing stand in your way. By focusing all of your energy to the job at hand there is no time to get involved with the day-to-day problems that lead to stress. Office politics will become trivial because you simply don't have the time for them.

Procrastination

Our parents taught us never to put off until tomorrow anything that can be done today.

Sound advice. Always work on the things you don't want to do first, and leave the things that you'll enjoy doing until last. It is a little mental game that makes you work harder to get to the stuff you really enjoy, ending the day on a positive note.

Procrastination is often a symptom of not being able to make a decision. Go on, just do it. In the grand scale of life, most of the day-to-day decisions we make are rather trivial. Will they really matter in a few months' time? The more readily you are able to make a decision, the more confident you become. It's about dealing in the here and now. It's about finding your own voice.

Time zones

Set aside a block of time for each of your daily activities. Try to perform these tasks only during the time zones you have set. An example would be to plan to make all your phone calls between 10 and 11am and arrange all your meetings between 2 and 4pm. This helps to focus your mind and organise your day. These times don't have to be cast in concrete as there will always be exceptions to the rule, but it will eliminate distractions during the time you have set aside to complete your daily goals. Let everyone know the hours that you set aside for these activities and you will be surprised to find how much more you can get done during the day.

Our parents taught us never to put off until tomorrow anything that can be done today

10 essential items for every home office

Working from home is one of the best things I ever decided to do. I am inspired by my surroundings and appreciate that I am able to get some of my chores, like laundry, done at the same time. I generally work from my kitchen table because it is large and I can spread out all my work. It also means that at the end of the day I am forced to be tidy because it is shared space. You still need the office essentials to work successfully from home, so here is my top 10 list of what gets me through my working day.

Telephone
I use the mobile land line with a speakerphone, so that I am not confined to a single area.

Laptop computer
I like to take my office anywhere that inspires me. My laptop has a built-in fax modem, so that all I need is a telephone outlet for an instant office.

Comfortable chair
Make sure that the small of your back is well supported and the chair is positioned so that you look straight ahead at your computer when sitting upright, with your feet flat on the floor and your knees at 90° to your body.

Good lighting
A desk light with a halogen bulb gives a natural, efficient task light.

Calculator
My electronic organiser is multi-functional. It is my diary, address book and calculator. All the information is downloaded daily onto my laptop so that I always have a back-up. The calculator has big numbers so that I can see them without my reading glasses – a definite plus.

Supply of fine-tip black pens and sharp pencils
I keep all my pens and pencils in a pot next to my computer. An electric pencil sharpener is a real treat, as I can't write with a blunt pencil.

Notebook
Decide upon a type of notebook you like and keep a supply handy. I use mine as a record of old ideas.

Clock
I am always conscious of the amount of time I have to do a task. Having a clock in sight keeps me on the straight and narrow.

Flowers/plants
Flowers and plants always inspire me. They make the space more personal and add oxygen to the air.

Stationery
Take stock of the items you use the most and make sure that you always have a good supply of them to hand.

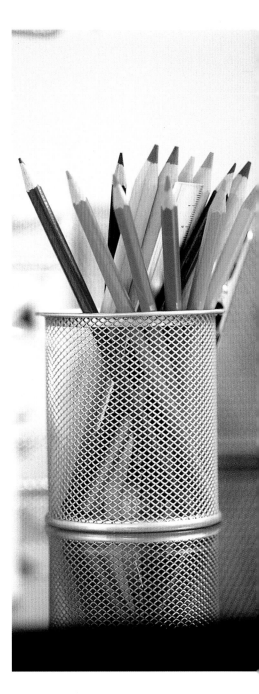

conquering the paper trail

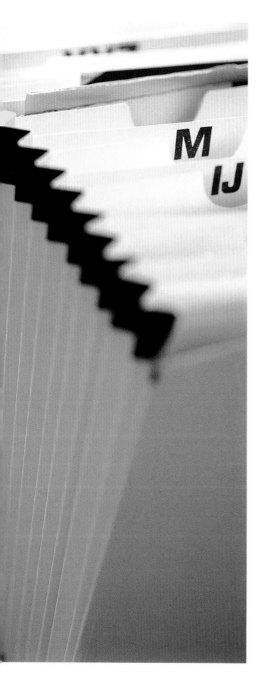

Talk more, write less

Some of us are in the habit of writing every little thing down. We pen a memo at the drop of a hat. I am not saying that keeping records isn't important, but sometimes we just do it out of habit. Have more conversations.

Keep a notebook

Never write things down on small scraps of paper. They will be all over the place and will get lost, which means that you will be frustrated. Have a notebook for recording any details that you need to keep. Label the outside of every notebook to remind you of what is inside and always date them.

Believe in technology

If you back up your computer daily onto floppy disks, Zips or Jazz drives, you will have less paper, more memory for new files and less chaos. Do it daily.

Edit

Make it a rule to edit your papers every day. Start with the things that you receive that day, from letters to memos, and recycle anything that you don't need to keep. Utilise your decision-making skills.

Whenever you have something new to add to your files, check to see if there is anything that you can remove. If you don't look, the file will just continue to grow until it falls apart and you aren't able to find anything in it.

Delegate

Forward anything that should be dealt with by someone else – immediately. It will be no good to anyone if you keep hold of a document you don't need until the day before the deadline, when there will not be enough time for anyone else to deal with it satisfactorily.

Capture the important bits

Many of us keep old newspapers and magazines stacked up sky high. Go through them and rip out the relevant bits and keep them in notebooks by subject. It will make a handy personal reference library and getting rid of the rest will make you feel good.

File

Set up a good filing system that makes sense to you. Have a file for everything, clearly labelled by category, and file your papers every day. Do not allow miscellaneous papers to pile up. If you can't figure out what to do with something, why are you keeping it in the first place? Stacks of paper only remind us of all the things we haven't done, so if in doubt, file it in the bin.

Put things in storage

Papers that you don't need but must retain for legal or other reasons should be put into long-term storage. Box them up and carefully label the outside so that you can easily get them when they are needed.

10 things to do before you leave the office

When you have finished your work, put it behind you. Do everything you can to bring closure to the day. Let your mind have the time to refresh and renew itself. Distance always gives you perspective.

Always back up your computer

Don't wait until disaster strikes. It just takes seconds.

Throw away or recycle all papers that you don't need

It will give you the opportunity to focus on the things that really matter.

Delegate

Go through your in-tray and delegate as much as possible. Pass things on before you leave the office. The only way to advance in life is to let go and be a good teacher.

Clear your desk of all clutter

It will give you a fresh start in the morning.

File all your papers

It always feels great to finish something. Filing things away gives you a sense of closure and accomplishment.

Spend time returning calls

You should always make the time to return phone calls on the same day. No one is that important that they can't take a few minutes to respond to a call.

Prioritise for tomorrow

Make a quick five-minute list of what you hope to achieve. You will immediately have your goals in front of you tomorrow.

Reflect on the day

Think about what you achieved and why. Think about the things that slipped through the cracks and deal with them first thing in the morning.

Say thank you

Make it a point to thank the people who have helped you during the day. It goes a very long way to making your job more enjoyable.

Save the environment

Turn off all your electrical appliances where possible. Check that there is paper in your fax machine, turn on your answer phone, if appropriate, and switch off the lights.

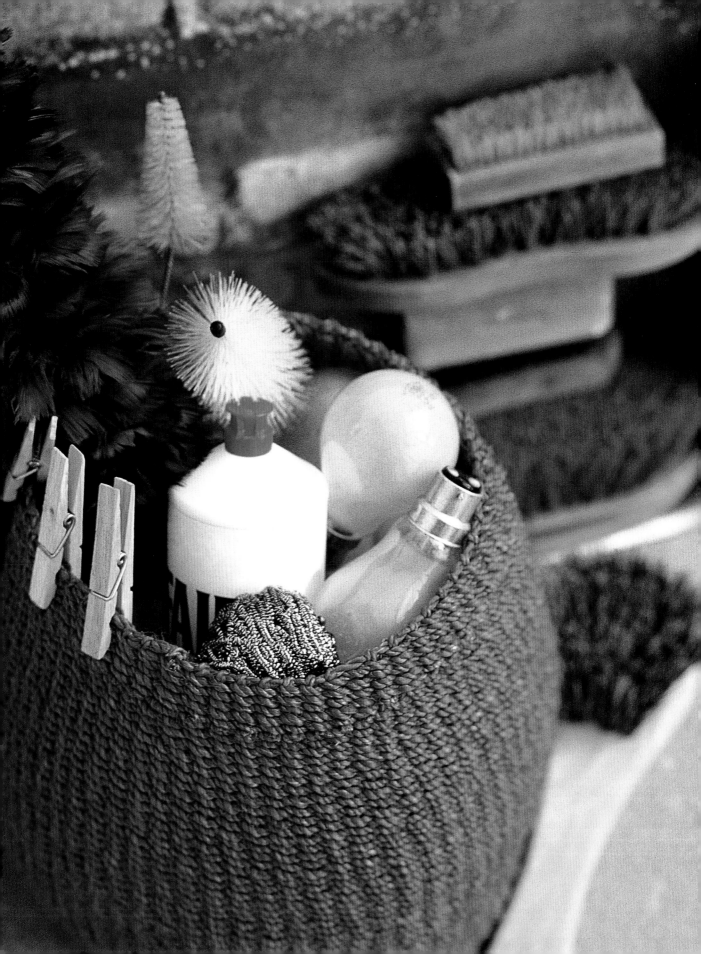

homework

I was once asked in an interview what I would do if my mother-in-law announced that she was 10 minutes away and my house was in utter chaos. I have to admit that I have occasionally thrown things into the downstairs cupboard on the arrival of an unannounced guest but, for the most part, my house is neat and tidy enough to receive guests at any time. I can't help it. I really am tidy.

But who needs the drama of trying to tidy up instantly? Doing the small things every day and getting everyone in the house to be responsible for themselves are much easier. Set the example. Make the small things part of your daily routine. Wipe out the bathroom sink every time you use it. Five seconds? Hang up your clothes whenever you change. Three minutes? Make your bed. Your

mother told you to do it and it is good advice. It's as simple as that. If these few things are done daily, your house will be generally tidy. Maybe not dust free and ready for inspection, but liveable in.

Bigger cleaning adventures need to be done periodically, some things with greater frequency than others. Make them part of the weekly, monthly or even seasonal routine and set aside the same time each week, month or half-year to clean so that you don't forget.

If you live in a shared house there have to be some rules for the common good and everyone should obey them. Think about the things that your parents taught you when you were a child. Do you practise them now or are you still rebelling? If you have children, what are you teaching them?

How clean your house needs to be depends on you. Some people can't live with a speck of dust – I have even heard of someone who employs a cleaner to wash her glasses every day. I just want my house to be relatively clean, with everything in its place and no papers lying about. I want it to look nice.

Pets are another responsibility and can present a cleaning challenge. We have two standard poodles, Sydney and Lola, who upon returning from the park every morning require at least a 15-minute clean-up. I wanted them and I gladly clean up after them. Remember who wanted the pet in your house!

The important thing to remember is that your house is your sanctuary. If it makes you happy, it's perfect for you and for anyone who is invited inside.

10 tips for instant tidiness

If the arrival of an unexpected guest would get your heart rate up without the benefit of aerobic exercise, try some emergency clean-up tips from American household specialist Mary Ellen Pinkham.

Look in the mirror

Check your appearance. Run a quick comb through your hair and put on a touch of lipstick. Your guests will look at you before they look at the state of your house.

Vacuum

If time allows, have a quick vacuum of the sitting room.

Fluff

Fluff up the all the pillows and cushions of the sofa.

Fool them with scent

Spray the living room with some pine furniture spray. It gives the appearance that everything has been thoroughly scrubbed.

Close doors

Limit the amount of rooms that you have to quickly tidy. Close the doors to all rooms except the one area in which you will entertain.

Clear the hallway

Get rid of all the junk on the floors and surfaces of both the hallway and the living room. Throw it all in a big box and hide it!

Dust

Spray some cleaner onto a duster and quickly go over the surfaces in the room in which you'll be sitting.

Smile

Open the door to your guests with a smile. Remember – they are here to visit you and not to inspect your home. Relax.

Get rid of the dishes

Clear the counters. Put everything in the dishwasher or oven. Give the surfaces a quick once-over with a sponge.

Check the bathroom

Get rid of any stray hairs in the sink. Check on your supply of toilet paper. Put out a new towel and throw anything on the floor in your laundry basket. If it is over-flowing, hide it in the shower and don't forget to pull the curtain.

easy cleaning

Make the chores described overleaf for each room part of a regular routine and forget about ever having to spend hours and hours cleaning.

Enlist the help of everyone in the house for the communal areas, where ground rules must apply, but don't get frustrated at the condition of anyone else's personal room, because it isn't yours and you aren't responsible for cleaning it. Communal living areas are the responsibility of everyone. Don't ever forget this fact and don't ever try to do everything, because you will always be frustrated.

Kids' rooms

Kids are another rule altogether. Teach your children well. Remember that everything they are taught now will remain with them. Set them an example and give them achievable goals.

- Teach them to make their bed every day.
- Make sure they can reach the rail in their closet and teach them to hang up their clothes when they have finished with them.
- Make a routine of putting toys away.

Larger tasks

There are certain cleaning chores that don't need to be done very regularly but should never be forgotten about. These are the tasks that should be undertaken every six months or once a year.

Spring ahead, Fall behind – things to do every six months

There is nothing like a change in the seasons to prompt a massive tidy. It always seems to me to symbolise a new beginning, and what better way than to start with refreshing your home?

Set aside a few hours of the weekend and only do one area of the house at a time. I like to start with the bedroom, as this is where I need to relax at the end of the day. When you've finished, treat yourself to something wonderful: a cup of coffee, a luxurious bubble bath, an hour sitting in your favourite chair listening to your favourite piece of music.

Yearly check-up

- Remove the limescale from everywhere that it appears.
- Have the rugs shampooed.
- Check the heating or air-conditioning systems.
- Have the chimneys swept.
- Clean all of your major appliances.
- Don't forget to clean the detergent dispensers in your washing and dishwashing machines.
- Remove the crumbs from the toaster.
- Go through all of your personal papers and throw away any that you no longer need.
- Spend a day putting photographs in albums.
- Call a friend you haven't spoken to in a while.

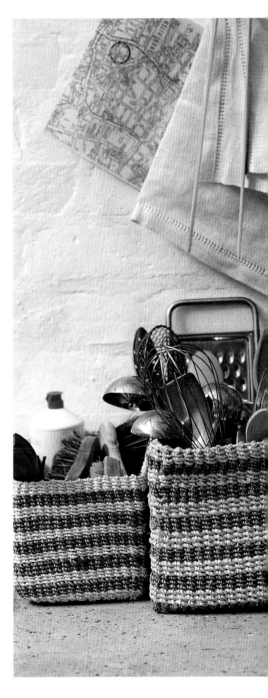

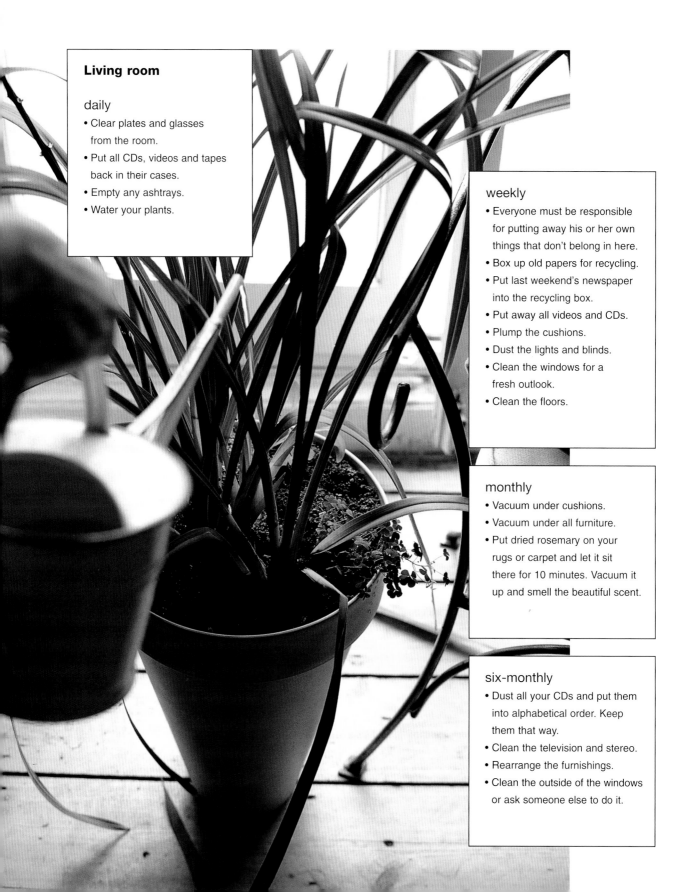

Living room

daily
- Clear plates and glasses from the room.
- Put all CDs, videos and tapes back in their cases.
- Empty any ashtrays.
- Water your plants.

weekly
- Everyone must be responsible for putting away his or her own things that don't belong in here.
- Box up old papers for recycling.
- Put last weekend's newspaper into the recycling box.
- Put away all videos and CDs.
- Plump the cushions.
- Dust the lights and blinds.
- Clean the windows for a fresh outlook.
- Clean the floors.

monthly
- Vacuum under cushions.
- Vacuum under all furniture.
- Put dried rosemary on your rugs or carpet and let it sit there for 10 minutes. Vacuum it up and smell the beautiful scent.

six-monthly
- Dust all your CDs and put them into alphabetical order. Keep them that way.
- Clean the television and stereo.
- Rearrange the furnishings.
- Clean the outside of the windows or ask someone else to do it.

Bathroom

daily

- Wipe out the bathroom sink after each use – it just takes a second and never turns into a big chore.
- Give the bath a good clean as soon as you step out of it.
- Wipe excess water from shower doors.
- Clean the toothpaste cap.
- Empty the wastepaper basket.

weekly

- Replace the toilet paper and make a note to buy more if you are running low.
- Clean the toilet.
- Wash the bathroom floor.
- Dust the shelves.
- Make sure you have clean, fresh towels.

monthly

- Clear out your bathroom cupboards and throw away whatever you really don't use.
- Give your mirrors a really good clean.
- Wash your bathroom rug.

six-monthly

- Get rid of old make-up and medicines.
- Polish all the hardware.
- Make your tiles sparkle.
- Wash or clean your curtains.
- Clean the shelves or cupboards.

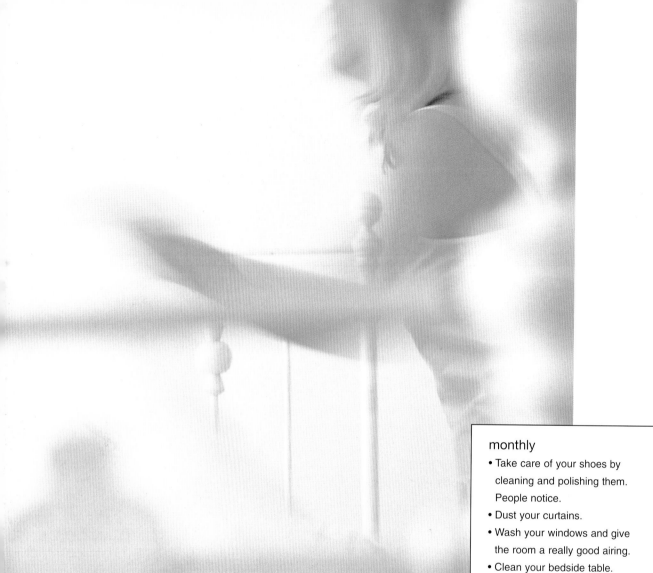

monthly
- Take care of your shoes by cleaning and polishing them. People notice.
- Dust your curtains.
- Wash your windows and give the room a really good airing.
- Clean your bedside table.

Bedroom

daily
- Make your bed.
- Hang up your clothes when you have finished wearing them.
- Take any glasses and cups into the kitchen.
- Put any unnecessary papers into a box for recycling.

weekly
- Put on clean sheets.
- Open the windows – even if it's raining.
- Vacuum the floor.
- Do the laundry.
- Make sure all your clothes are neatly folded and put away.
- Put flowers next to the bed.
- Water the plants.

six-monthly
- Edit your wardrobe and be honest.
- Give to charity what you really don't need.
- Throw the windows wide open regardless of the temperature.
- Turn the mattress.
- Wash your mattress cover if you have one.
- Change to a thinner or thicker duvet depending on the season.

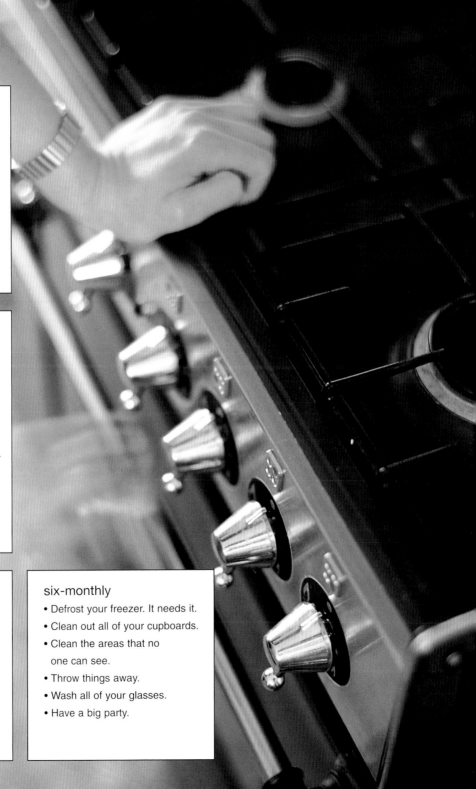

Kitchen

daily

- Always wash the dishes. Always!
- Empty the dishwasher.
- Clear and clean all the work surfaces.
- Put everything that can be recycled into the correct boxes.

weekly

- Bin anything that is past its use-by date.
- Give the inside of your refrigerator a good wipe-down.
- Make sure that the ice cube trays are full.
- Empty and clean the rubbish bin.
- Dust everything that is visible.
- Dust everything else!
- Clean your floors.

monthly

- Scrub the pots and pans.
- Clean the oven. Don't forget.
- Clean under the kitchen sink.
- Clean out the cutlery drawer.
- Polish any silverware.
- Take your items for recycling to your local recycling bins.

six-monthly

- Defrost your freezer. It needs it.
- Clean out all of your cupboards.
- Clean the areas that no one can see.
- Throw things away.
- Wash all of your glasses.
- Have a big party.

getting on top of laundry

I have to tell the truth here. Although I do laundry all the time I'm not very good at it. Even though I sort through everything my whites are never very white. I think I've got the hang of it all through my research and, hand over heart, I am going to get better. One way around the problem is to do less of it.

I bet that most of us feel that we spend too much time doing laundry. The answer is that we probably do. Sometimes it's just easier to throw something in the laundry basket than to hang it up. Confess. It's true, isn't it? Always remember that eventually you will have to fold or hang it, so you might as well get into the habit of hanging things up when you've finished wearing them and launder less often. It's better for your clothes and saves you time.

Laundry know-how

This is the important bit. Read the little print on the label to check the care instructions before you buy an item of clothing, and before you launder it, to avoid disasters. We don't really want to give our children, or their dolls, our best jumpers. Care labels are required by law, so before you buy, make sure your garment has one attached. Each label should have a variety of symbols, which give you the information you need about how to wash, dry and iron the garment. If any of the symbols are crossed through it means the garment shouldn't be given that treatment.

 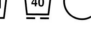 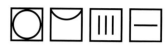

Washing

The washing symbol resembles a tub and shows the temperature that should be used. If the tub has lines underneath this usually means that the garment should be washed on a cycle with a gentle spin. Two lines underneath the tub means wash on a cycle that has a delicate spin. A hand in the washing tub, you guessed it, means to hand-wash with lukewarm water. A circle represents dry cleaning, although it may be possible for you to hand-wash any garment that states it should be dry-cleaned (see page 66).

Bleaching

The international symbol for bleach is a triangle. It means that bleach can be used on the garment, if necessary. If 'Cl' is written inside the triangle this means that chlorine bleach can be used on the garment.

Drying

A square represents drying. If the square has a circle inside it this represents a tumble-dryer. If the circle inside the square has two dots it means tumble-dry on medium to high heat. A circle inside the square with one dot indicates that the garment should be dried on low heat. If the symbol looks like an envelope or a hanging line across the square it means line-dry. Three vertical lines in the square means hang wet to drip dry and a horizontal line in the middle of the square means dry on a flat surface.

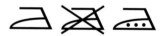

Ironing

It really looks like an iron. Three dots on the symbol mean the maximum setting on hot, as used for cotton or linen. Two dots mean that you should iron with medium heat. One dot means iron on a low setting.

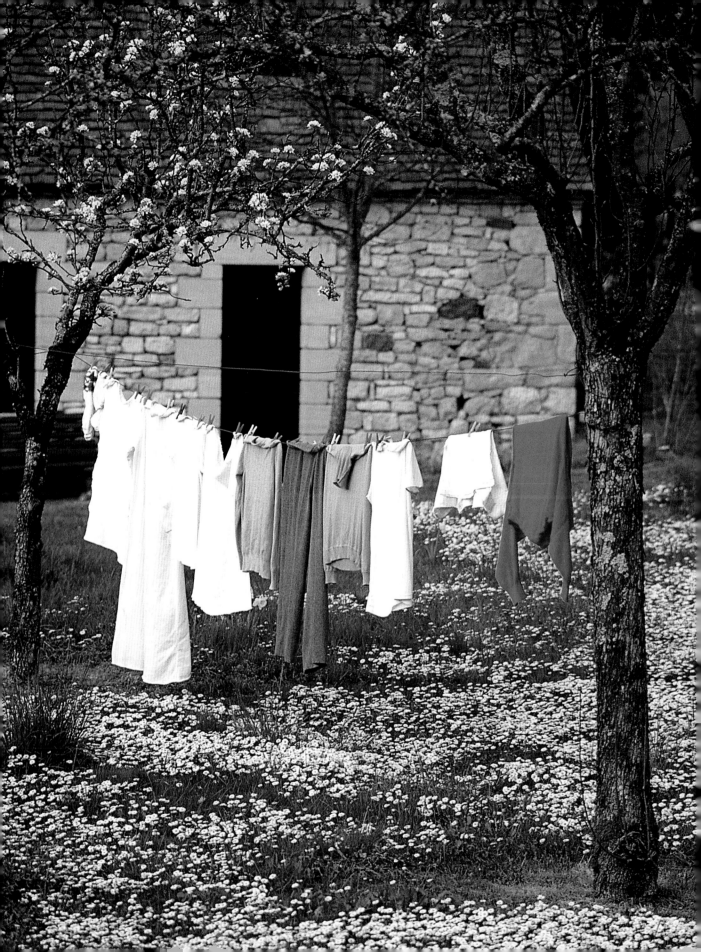

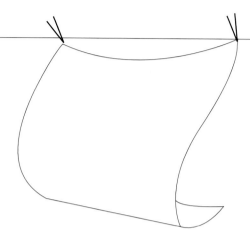

Dry-cleaning

Some items require dry-cleaning, but take care not to clean them too often as it is really hard on the fabric. If the garment has become wrinkled and the wrinkles won't hang out, send it off to be pressed rather than cleaned. It saves money and wear and tear on your clothes.

The dry-cleaning symbol is a circle. Although every garment with a dry-cleaning symbol can possibly be hand-washed, you will do so against the manufacturer's advice and will be responsible if things go wrong. Exercise caution. Any garment with colours that will run, details such as pleats or beading or is tailored with padding must be sent to the cleaner's. There are three different letters that may appear in the dry-cleaning symbol circle – P, A or F – which indicate the chemicals that the cleaner should or should not use. Don't bother yourself with the chemistry of it. Just use a really good dry-cleaner.

Sorting your laundry

In an ideal world, you would sort your laundry by colour, by fabric and by how dirty it is. You would probably spend 30 years of your life washing. Use your head. Don't mix lights and whites with darks ,because you know what will happen. Wash items that require bleach together and don't do it in a hurry. One black sock and disaster strikes.

If a garment is marked 'wash separately' it means that the dye could run and ruin your other clothing. Give it a miss in your next load. This colour-run problem can last for the life of the garment, not just the first few washes. Don't mix towels or anything fluffy with items that are not – fluff can take a long time to remove.

Before you begin

Always check all the pockets of the clothes for chewing gum,tissues, tickets etc., or you may find an unpleasant sight when you open your machine. If anything requires mending – loose buttons or tears – these will only get worse in the wash, so repair them now. Keep a sewing box with needles already threaded with basic colours and this won't seem such a chore.

Button everything up, keep zips zipped and turn heavy items that might bobble inside out. We all know about sock heaven. To keep your socks back on an earthly plane, put them in a mesh bag and don't worry about it. Better yet, keep the mesh bag in your laundry hamper and throw them in when you get undressed.

Pre-soak or spot anything that is heavily soiled, taking care to read the label for colour-fastness. Always do a test on an area of the garment that will not be seen before you spot-clean.

Drying

Clothes do not have to be dried in a machine. If you haven't got one or just prefer to hang them outside to dry, try giving them an extra spin in your washing machine to remove most of the excess moisture. Gently reshape your garments before hanging them up to dry. You can avoid all that time-consuming ironing of many clothes by taking this extra step prior to drying. If you don't have a line outside, string up one in your bathroom or laundry room. Hanging creates fewer wrinkles than placing them on a rack.

If you do use a tumble-dryer, clean the lint filter often. Don't over-dry your clothes – it is harder on the fabric and makes them more difficult to iron. Take them out of the dryer while they are less than bone dry and hang them promptly. If you have over-dried permanent-press clothing, return them to the dryer with a damp towel and put them through a low cycle, remove and then iron on a low setting.

Shake, rattle and roll

Put small items in the bottom of the machine and the bulkier items on top. Set the appropriate water temperature and cycle and add your detergent. Read the instructions. Every detergent is different. Add the right amount for the job at hand. Add required bleach and fabric softeners if your machine dispenses them automatically, making certain that the products can safely be mixed. Don't let clothing sit in the washing machine when the cycle is complete. Wrinkles will set in and the longer the clothes sit, the more likely they are to mildew.

accidents happen

Accidents will always happen – just accept it. Laugh about it. If the stain doesn't come out the world won't end.

Stain removal

You need to act quickly. Blot a spillage with an absorbent cloth immediately. Do a test in a hidden area first to make sure that it will not make another stain, then use a little stain-remover or water, according to the type of stain. Keep an old toothbrush handy and pour the stain remover onto the brush before treating the stain. Be patient.

Have a stain-removal kit in your laundry room with the following items: acetone, automatic dishwasher liquid, bicarbonate of soda, bleach, colour remover, enzyme pre-soak, glycerine (available from the chemist), hydrogen peroxide 3%, pre-wash stain remover, rubbing alcohol and white vinegar.

The following remedies are for washable items only. If the item needs to be dry-cleaned take it to the cleaner's as soon as possible.

Alcoholic beverages

Soak the stained item in a solution of cold water and 30ml glycerine. Add 240ml white vinegar to a sink filled with cold water to rinse the soaked item.

Blood

If the stain is fresh use salt or hydrogen peroxide; if it has set, use an enzyme-based stain remover and cold water.

Fruit stains

Mix equal parts of vinegar, water and dishwashing soap. Pour onto the stain. Allow to stand, then rinse with cold water.

Grass

Dab the stain with an enzyme-based stain remover or apply rubbing alcohol, then rinse with cold water.

Grease

Sprinkle talcum powder onto the stain and allow to dry. Brush the powder off, then launder the item as usual.

Gum

Put the item in the freezer until the gum is hard. Scrape off the gum and let the item come to room temperature. Add lighter fluid to a damp cloth and rub into the gum stain. Launder as usual.

Ink

Apply rubbing alcohol with a clean cloth.

Lipstick/make-up

Dab a non-oily make-up remover onto the stain, then launder as usual.

Marker pen

Run cold water over the stain until most of the ink is removed. Put the fabric on a paper towel and pour rubbing alcohol on the stain.

Wine

Use a generous amount of soda water.

Carpets and rugs

Time is of the essence with carpet stains, as the longer the stain remains, the more difficult it is to remove. Blot liquid stains with a soft, white absorbent material such as a towel.

If solid materials have fallen onto the carpet, scrape them away using a blunt object (such as a spatula) to avoid damaging the fibres and then vacuum up as much as possible. Never scrub or brush a stain as this can cause it to set.

Keep to hand several types of carpet cleaners. Always check for colour-fastness by applying a few drops to each colour in the carpet. Then press a clean white towel or serviette to the area and check that no colour has been transferred to the towel. If it has, try another cleaning agent.

Always start from the outside of the stain and work inwards to prevent the stain from getting larger. Apply the removal agent to the towel and gently dab onto the stain. Keep adding the agent to the towel and continue with the process as long as the stain remains. Be patient. It can be a long process.

If the first agent doesn't remove the stain, try another. When the stain has gone, remove the agent from the carpet using the same procedure but with fresh water.

Gently blot the area until it is dry, using a clean white towel. As one towel becomes saturated, place another over the affected area until it is dry.

10 best items for chemical-free cleaning

Chamois cloth
Great for washing windows and polishing cars. It is absorbent, cleans and polishes.

Lemon oil
Typically used as a furniture polish, it is the best cleaner for stainless steel, removing fingerprints and keeping it looking highly polished.

White vinegar
A bowl of white vinegar left out in a smoky room will absorb the smell. It is also a great window cleaner used with newspapers and is an effective stain remover for most fabrics.

Automatic dishwashing powder
Even if you don't have a dishwasher, use the powder to remove the rings around your bathtub and a multitude of other stains.

Long-handled feather duster
Don't overstretch yourself, unless your cleaning is part of an exercise routine. Get at all the cobwebs in the most out of the way places.

Spray bottles
Keep a few good-quality spray bottles filled with rubbing alcohol and water. Make sure to label them on the outside. They are quick and versatile and will come in handy throughout your house.

Rubber gloves
Your hands show your age. Protect them when using all household cleaners or when soaking in water.

Sponge mop/pail
Try to find a pail that has two compartments – one for soapy water and one to rinse. It saves both time and effort.

Steel wool
Use steel wool pads sparingly, as they are abrasive and wear down the surface you are cleaning. But they are essential for removing some difficult stains in the kitchen.

Vacuum cleaner
The best vacuums don't require bags, as there is no loss of suction and you never have to worry about changing an over-full bag. If you have a conventional vacuum, always buy spare bags.

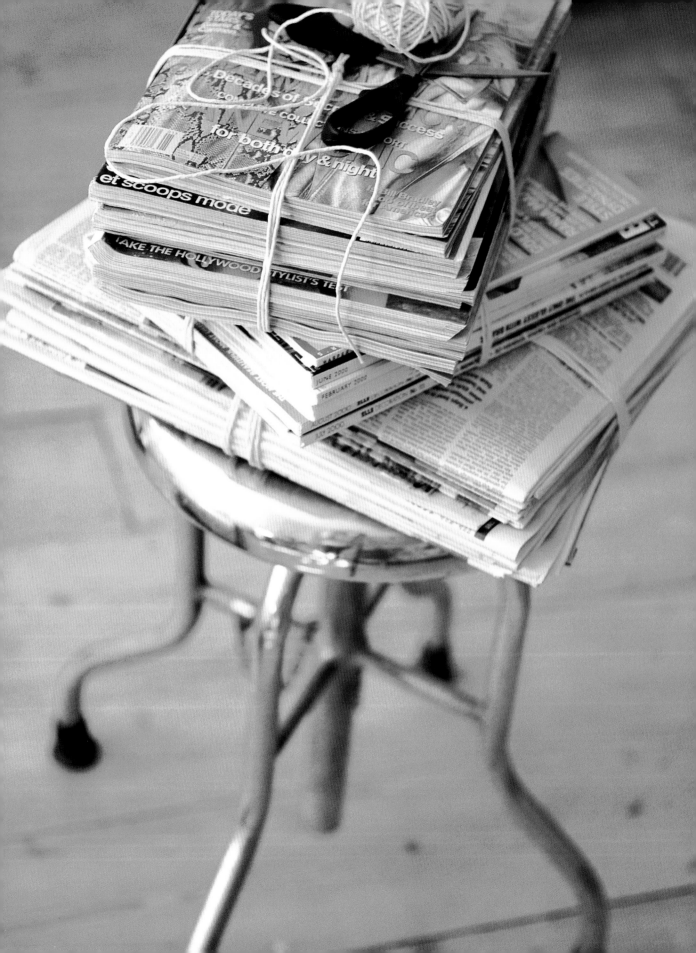

clearing the clutter

What is it that makes us have the urge to hoard so many things and then have such a difficult time parting with them when they have outlived whatever usefulness they may once have had? Are we hanging on to old memories? Is it the fear that we will throw something away that could have a dramatic impact on our lives? Maybe it is just an inability to know where to begin.

Focus on the here and now

According to Feng Shui expert Karen Kingston, when we hold on to old papers we do not allow ourselves to create space for new ideas to come into our lives. Think about your house. Are there stacks of newspapers and magazines sitting in a corner? Bills stuffed into drawers around the house? Book shelves filled to the brim leaving no room for your current inspirations? Photographs piled in boxes collecting dust that you haven't looked at in years? Let the energy and new ideas flow by ridding yourself of a past that is no longer relevant. Start afresh and open yourself to new ideas. This is how we learn and grow. Start today. Lighten up and feel free.

Well read

Step by step, begin to rid yourself of the weight. Start with your books. They have helped you to develop your views on life. They have inspired you and been there to comfort you. Feng Shui disciples would say that when you have too many books on your book shelf you become set in your ways. Are you becoming set in your ways?

Go through all of the books you have in your home. Really assess them. Those you will never read, no longer have a use for – like old textbooks – or have just outgrown should be donated to a charity shop or library. Give some of your favourite books to your friends. Share your wisdom. Keep some of those books that truly reflect who you are now, but make space for who you will become.

Make it a rule of the household that newspapers are recycled daily and that magazines can only stay during the life of the issue. Make ideas books. When you read through magazines and newspapers, take out the information that inspires you and save it in your own personal reference system. Even your ideas books should be edited every so often to make way for new inspiration. Yesterday's news is old hat.

Photographic memory

Can you feel the blocked energy flowing? How often do you look at all of your old photographs, stuffed in drawers, shoe boxes and albums?

Not often, if you are like me. I am going to begin today to get rid of the past and keep only those memories that I want to keep with me. I will vow to put lots of my photographs in picture frames – which can be placed around the house – and the rest in albums, to make them more accessible both to myself and to visitors.

The same is true for sentimental journeys from your past. Don't feel guilty about getting rid of all those letters and birthday cards that you never look at. Keep the ones that truly mean something and clear the way for memories yet to be made. Don't wallow in sad memories of the past. Move on with life and enjoy the present.

Save the planet

So many items in the modern home, from paper and cardboard to bottles and tins, can be recycled. It's the only way to go and gives you a positive reason to clear away the inessentials from every area of your life. Load all your old paper, plastic, bottles and cans into boxes and take them down to the local recycling bins whenever you need to. Check with your local council which materials they can recycle – you may find that even the majority of your kitchen waste can be recycled to make a wonderfully rich compost.

Knowing that you are helping the environment is often enough motivation for you to edit all your papers regularly. Most forms of paper can be recycled, although they should be separated into colours and types before being placed into the correct recycling bin. Again, check the procedure with your council.

paperwork

We are all bombarded almost every day with junk mail, letters, newspapers, magazines and bills. We need to sort through it all. Piles of papers hidden in every drawer and cupboard are a constant reminder that you need to take control of the situation.

Important documents

We all have essential documents that prove who we are and what we own, including passport, birth certificate, insurance policies, vehicle registration details, wills, share certificates and licences. A copy of all credit cards should also be kept with these papers. All of the above can be replaced, but only after a certain amount of trouble and time.

Ideally these documents should be kept inside a fire-retardant box or cabinet for maximum security and protection. It is advisable that with items such as insurance policies, wills and share certificates, the originals should be stored in a bank safe-deposit box or with your solicitor. Keep a copy of everything for your files in case you need to access the details quickly.

Finances

As I am sure most of us have found on occasion, banks and credit card companies can and do make mistakes. It is always best to get into the habit of checking your statements when they arrive and then, once you are happy that they are correct, filing them chronologically. I find that the best method is to use an accordion file for the year, with a pocket for each month.

I don't know why we feel the need to save statements for years and years. Ask yourself how many times you have ever needed to get information from your oldest statements. For Inland Revenue and house-buying purposes you should keep six years' worth of statements and receipts, but anything older than that really should go.

File all but the current year in sturdy cardboard boxes, one for each year, clearly marked on the outside. Store them in an out-of-the-way location, such as a damp-proofed loft, basement, cupboard or under the bed. If you need them they can be accessed quickly but they won't take up space.

Pay your bills when they arrive.

Once you have checked the bill, make out the cheque – even if it isn't yet due – and write the date that it must be posted on the envelope. Keep the statement on file and the envelope in a position where you will be reminded to post it on the right date.

Warrantees and instructions

Designate one file or drawer in your home for all instruction manuals or warrantees. After years of owning a video machine, I still need to refer to the instructions from time to time. You will also sometimes need to use the registration number to report a fault. It is wise to affix the purchase record inside the manual for proof of purchase.

All the other stuff

Ruthlessly go through every paper in your office or hiding place and chuck out everything you don't need. Take as much as you can to the recycling bins. Reply to letters the day they arrive. You won't have a nagging feeling that there is always something you have to do if you do it in the present. Lighten up and let your soul fly.

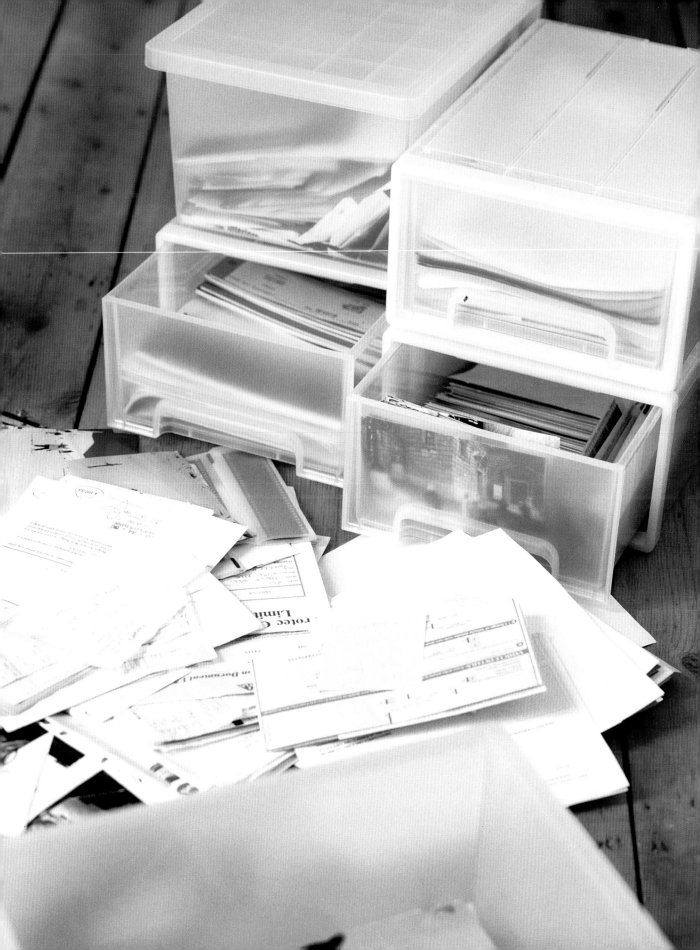

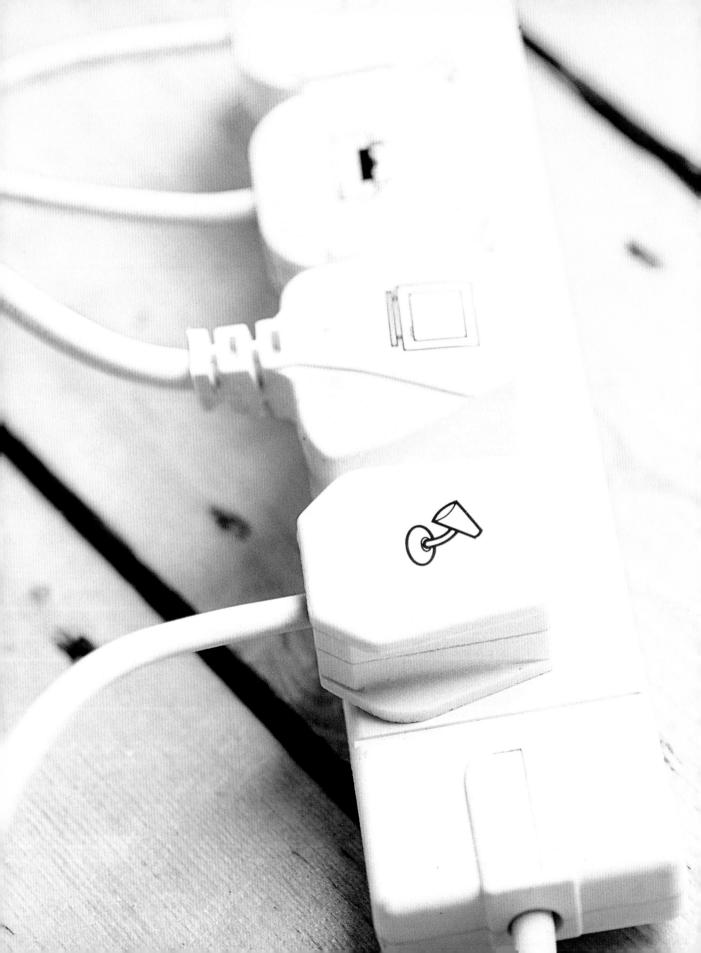

become a media mogul

Watching videos or listening to your favourite tunes is supposed to be entertaining, right? If frustration sets in because things aren't working properly or sound a little strange, it can be a pain not a pleasure. But a quick recap of the basics can banish your technical problems for ever.

Get to grips with it

Isn't it at least partly true that when we finally get our new electronic goods home – usually after a lengthy period of research and decision-making – we are so desperate to get it all set up that we don't actually read the instructions that are enclosed with it? Everything just comes out of its box and is plugged in wherever seems most appropriate.

Many a frustration is the result of a basic lack of knowledge about our electrical toys. Somewhere there are full instructions that tell you how to make each of them do what you want them to. Do you know what happened to the operating manual after the initial rush to unpack? If you can find it, get it out and go through the step-by-step operating procedures. Learn them, so that you won't get stuck when you are in a hurry. Knowledge is the key to success.

Take a few minutes to gather together your instruction manuals for everything you have in the house, then keep them all in the same place. A file marked 'equipment' would do the trick. They will always be easy to find.

Cable control

Get in control of all the cables that are attached to your electrical equipment. Put a sticky label on each cable so that you know what it does and where the other end needs to be plugged in. It will be a massive help if something goes wrong or if you want to move your equipment around. Also, there will be no danger of turning off the fish filter when you meant to turn off the toaster. Get plugged in.

Film

Keep track of what you have in your video/dvd library and you won't ever go searching for a blank tape to record over. Get a small notebook and some sticky labels. Label each tape or disk with a number on the outside of the cassette and on the box and set aside a few pages in the notebook for each numbered tape. Always keep a pen or pencil in the notebook. If you don't have any idea what is on the tapes, you will have to go through them one by one. You will then know what you have and what you are willing to record over. Every time you reuse a tape, amend your notebook accordingly by removing the old entry and listing the new one, along with the date if necessary.

Always put the tapes back in their correct box. It keeps your collection tidy and organised and will also stop dust from getting into the tape and ruining your machine.

Music

Work out which type of storage you prefer for your music. It will mainly depend on how many tapes, CDs and records that you have. Cassette racks and CD racks can hold up to 100 items and often have a few spaces for doubles. Keep them in alphabetical order, as this will limit the amount of time it takes to find the music that you instantly want to hear.

If you are a real music collector, store your collection in boxes, with a separate box for each music category. Place things alphabetically in the boxes for ease of reference. Remember when you had to do this kind of ordering as a child, to practise your alphabet? It gives your brain a quick workout and will enable you to go through your entire collection to see what you have and what you are still missing from your 'wish list'.

Make sure to edit your collection. If there are things that you never listen to any more, give them to a friend or take them to a second-hand shop and make enough money to buy something that you really want. Don't hold on to them. Our tastes change.

perfect pets

If I had to live without my dogs I would find life much less interesting. They bring such energy, warmth and laughter to every day. They are the reason that I take time every morning to walk in the park and subsequently clear my mind of work and any other worries. They are part of my family.

Instinctive behaviour

All animals have natural instincts. How we adapt these instincts to our living arrangements dictates how well our animals fit in with our lifestyle. Animals require the basics of food and shelter. Most of them also require human companionship. Be really clear in your mind that you are able to give these unconditionally before you decide to bring a pet into your life.

Research the characteristics of the pet you choose – don't rely on a pet store or breeder. Read some books. Talk to a veterinary surgeon. Never make a spur-of-the-moment decision. A pet really is for life! Think about your schedule and how much time you will be able to devote to your pet. Dogs require lots of human interaction and lots of exercise. The trouble begins when animals are alone and bored. Cats are more independent and can be happy on their own, although they like company sometimes. Animals that live in cages or tanks need less personal interaction and can often be left alone for periods of time as long as they are fed.

Leader of the pack

You are supposed to be the master. Top dog. Always remember this. Teach your pet the rules of the house. Dogs and cats require their own territory. Wherever this may be in your house, always keep any bedding and toys in this location. Train dogs to go to their basket on command. Practise this daily and when you really want them out of the way, they will obey. Every now and then sit in their spot. It reinforces the fact that you are the boss.

If you have pets, keeping the house fresh smelling and clean is the greatest challenge. For pets that shed, it is essential to groom them regularly. This means brushing them every few days to remove the undercoat of hair. For cats it is essential because if they groom themselves they can develop hairballs that cause them to choke. The more you remove by brushing, the less likely they are to be ill. Did you know that the simple act of grooming or patting your pet can reduce blood pressure? Just what the doctor ordered!

House-training cats to use a litter tray and dogs to go outside is the single most important thing you will do. Cats are quick to learn and will get the knack of it in a few days' time. With dogs it can take longer. As puppies, take them for frequent walks outdoors, especially just after a meal. Always praise them for getting it right. Never scold them for making a mistake. If you

catch them in the act, quickly get them outdoors so they understand the association. Accidents will occasionally happen with all pets. To make sure they do not repeat their performance, neutralise the odour with an enzyme cleaner.

Companion for life

Do unto pets as you would do unto yourself. Groom them. Keep them clean. Wash their dishes. Give them fresh water all the time. Feed them the best food available. This will reinforce their dependency on you and will keep them obedient. The rewards definitely outweigh any hassle. Just the wag of a tail, a purr, a lick, can make the world right. A companion that is always there for you can reduce the stresses of life to insignificance. I highly recommend it.

The rewards definitely outweigh any hassle. Just the wag of a tail, a purr, a lick, can make the world right.

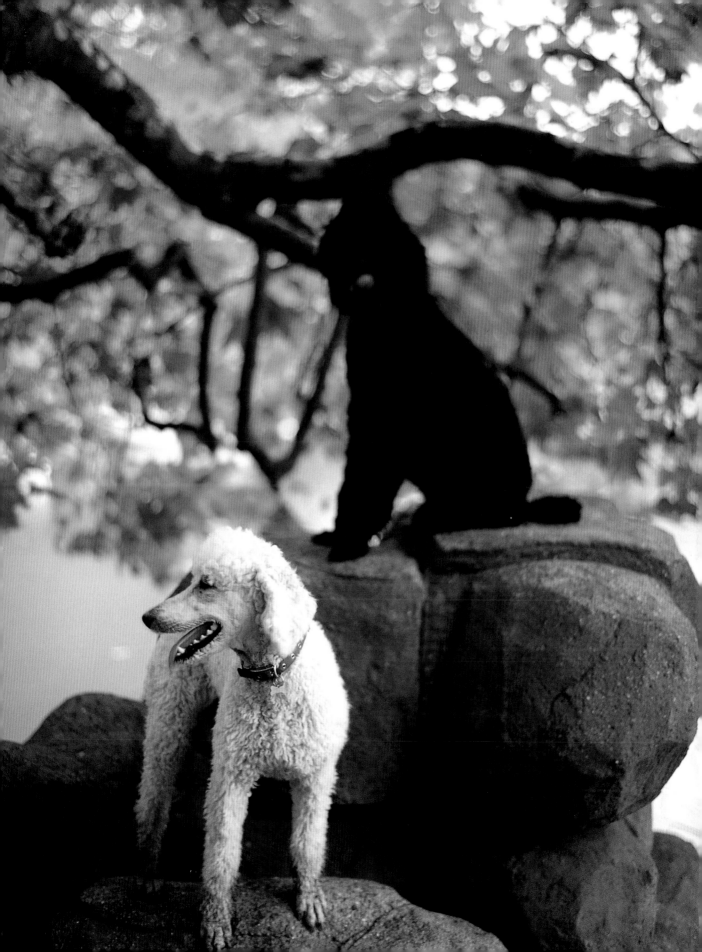

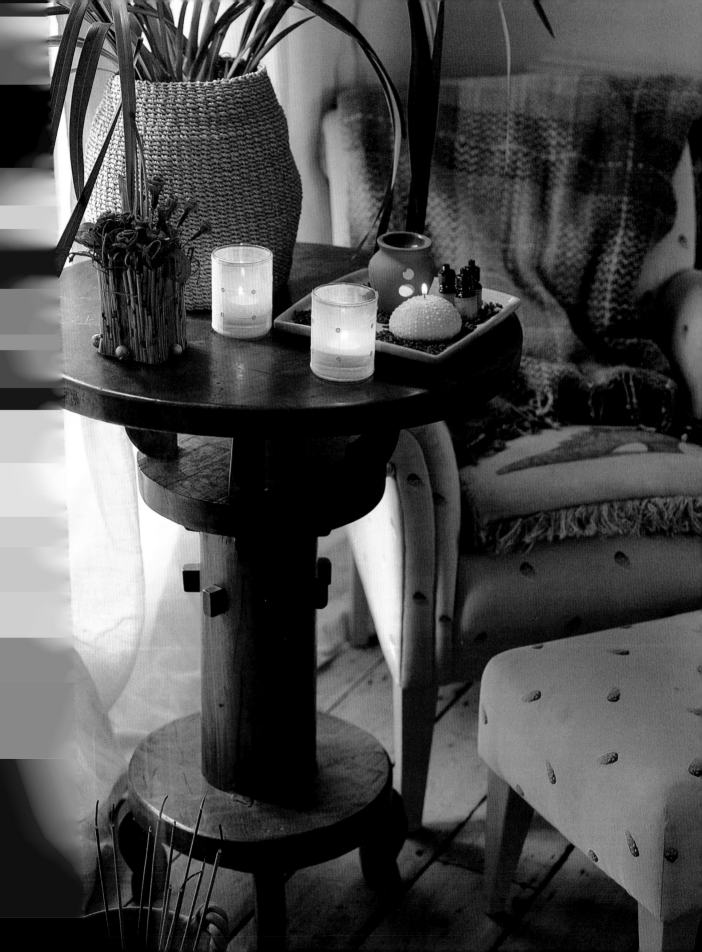

sanctuary

"Have nothing in your house that you do not know to be useful or believe to be beautiful." WILLIAM MORRIS

If you are happy with your surroundings you are fortunate, as your home truly is your sanctuary, a place where you can be totally yourself.

My home is very important to me. I smile every day at the colours in my kitchen. I am surrounded by mementoes of family and friends in America. I love to flop in my bargain chair that I brought with me from America and have a glass of wine. I enjoy my space.

If you are not happy with your home, you need to begin to make it your own. Take note of the quote by William Morris; usefulness and beauty are a great starting point in deciding what is really important to you in your home.

Whether single, in a couple or a family, your home displays your true self. A space that feels both personal and homely enables you to be comfortable with yourself, whether on your own or interacting with others. Your special sanctuaries are your bedroom and bathroom – the two most personal areas of your home. What do they say about you? Do you feel special and pampered in them?

Think about which area of the house is most important to you and start there. Personalise it. Surround yourself with things that feel good. If you love to read, stack books against a wall for decor and accessibility. If music is your passion, make the sound system a main feature.

Ensure that you have all the basics necessary for contentment. Make a list of the items you can't live without in each room. If you realise you don't have something, aspire to it.

Light and colour affect our mood. A bright, sunny day with the light coming in through the windows is bliss. Bright colours boost energy and soft colours are serene; different zones for different moods. How do the lighting and colour in your house affect your mood?

Kids and pets create special demands on our living space and require care and attention. What are your children's favourite activities? To develop their creativity give them a special area which will be theirs alone. Mark out a territory for your pet. That is their natural instinct. Indulge them.

Think about your vision of sanctuary. What makes you feel special? Take small steps to get you there, room by room. Enter into the fantasy of a perfect home. Enjoy yourself.

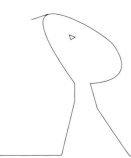

happy communal living

Living together happily requires that no one person feels that they are doing more than their fair share to keep the house running smoothly. This can be tricky, because, as individuals, we all have different standards and levels of expectation.

To get it right, everyone has to agree to a house standard – the basic level of cleanliness in the common areas of the home that will make you all happy and comfortable. Setting the standard leaves no room for any confusion.

Personal space is just that – personal. With the exception of children, who need to be taught to be tidy, adults should live as they wish. Don't interfere with what anyone else is doing and you won't be unhappy. This is a big lesson. Work at getting the balance and you will indeed be a happier person.

Show and tell

To begin, everyone needs to make a list, room by room, of all the things that they feel need to be done. Start when you walk in the door and go through all the rooms that you share. Sit down and have a group meeting and make sure that you listen to what each individual feels is important to them.

Once you have agreed on the basics, write them all down and keep them where everyone can see them. The list should be broken down into two sections – what each individual must do as part of their daily routine and specific weekly jobs that need to be done. The more that is completed daily, the less to worry about weekly.

It works for me

I always believe that if everything has a home and is kept there, your house will look tidy and liveable. It may not be spotless, but I can live with that.

The things that make me happy when done daily are:
- Hanging up coats as soon as you walk in the door.
- Putting all personal belongings in your room when you arrive home.
- Picking up papers or post and dealing with them immediately.
- Cleaning up your dishes when you are finished with them.
- Running the dishwasher.
- Emptying the dishwasher.
- Putting away food when you have finished with it.
- Always replacing the water in the ice cube tray.
- Cleaning work surfaces in the kitchen.

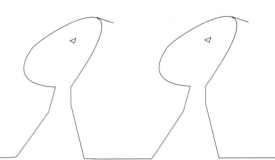

- Emptying the rubbish when the bin is full.
- Replacing the bin liner.
- Putting CDs/tapes away when you have finished with them.
- Turning off lights and electrical equipment when you have finished.

I'm sure that there are many more things that may be important to you. Get the daily chores right and you will never be angry or unhappy when you get home in the evening.

The big stuff

Weekly chores are the bigger cleaning jobs in the house such as vacuuming, mopping, dusting, changing bedlinens and doing the laundry. Decide as a group who will be responsible for each job and when it will be done. Try to do it at the same time each week and it will become part of your routine.

Change the jobs weekly if that's the way it works best for you or get everyone to pick the one they like the most and make it their permanent household job.

Setting the stage for personal development

If you have children, this is the time to teach them about sharing. Every child needs to learn that we all have a responsibility to join in for the common good of achieving a particular goal. It is an important lesson and the earlier you teach it the better.

Let them earn their pocket money every week by successfully doing their household chores. It will have a lasting impact on their development and attitudes towards sharing, working and responsibility and will make them better adults. Their future partners or flatmates will thank you for it!

Above and beyond

If your individual standards are higher than the groups, then by all means do what you have to do to feel happy in your own home. Clean until everything sparkles. Hopefully, other people's participation in achieving the basics will make your job easier. Don't ever get angry because you are going the extra cleaning mile on your own – it's your choice!

10 things to make your house more homely

Think about what it felt like to go back to the house you lived in as a child after you moved out on your own. It might be a smell or an old, worn-out armchair by the fireplace that evoked feelings of being nurtured and protected. Think about the things that you loved most about where you lived when you were growing up. Make your house a home by adding some of the elements that comforted you when you were young. Update them to suit your own personal style.

Cushions
Soften the lines of a sofa or chair with cushions. They are a great way to experiment with colours and patterns, and can also help support your back or be used as a pillow for a quick snooze

Candles
Candles have always been used in sacred spaces. They add soul to any room. Try spending an evening in a room lit only by candles. The room will immediately be transformed into a magical, warm space that seems to be made for relaxing. Bliss.

Photographs
Remind yourself of your happiest memories with framed photographs. Group them together on a wall or use them on tables and mantelpieces. Make it a point to look at them and think happy thoughts.

Blanket/throw
Keeping a lovely blanket or throw on your sofa makes it feel more inviting. Snuggle up inside it to read your favourite book or to watch television.

Rugs
Something as simple as adding a rug can make a huge difference to how a room feels. Put them on wooden floors, tiles or even on top of fitted carpets to give some character to your space. They don't have to be new. Spend some time looking for just the right one.

Perfect chair
Everyone should have a chair to call his or her own: a chair that envelops you and feels as if it were designed for you alone. Think of it as your throne, as a place where you can go and be in control of your own life. You don't have to buy the first chair that you see. Sit in it for a while. If it feels right, it will become an old friend.

Scent
Our sense of smell carries with it lasting associations with events from our past. I will always associate the smell of cloves with my first trip to the dentist. Try as I may, it won't go away. Adding fragrance to your home can help your mind and body to relax. Essential oils, potpourri, scented candles and fresh flowers are all great ways to lift your spirits.

Table lamps
Choose a more intimate lighting scheme and soften the edges of your room. The right table lamp can cast a lovely glow and create a more intimate space. Use a lamp shade with warm tones and team it with a frosted low-watt bulb for a subtle effect.

Plants
My mother always had African violets in our house when I was growing up. For me, plants give immediate warmth to any room in the house. Use them to add colour or to shade a window. Grow living herbs in front of your kitchen window. They are something you must nurture for them to flourish. They let the world know that nature-loving people reside inside your home.

Baskets
Many baskets are still hand-made from natural materials – which means that each of them is unique – so I always prefer to buy these. Every culture throughout time has used baskets to both carry and store things. They come in all sizes, shapes and colours and can be used to store most things. Try a big log basket by the fireplace, or a smaller one by the side of your favourite chair to hold your magazines. Each basket, as well as offering useful storage just where you need it, will give your house an added touch of warmth and colour.

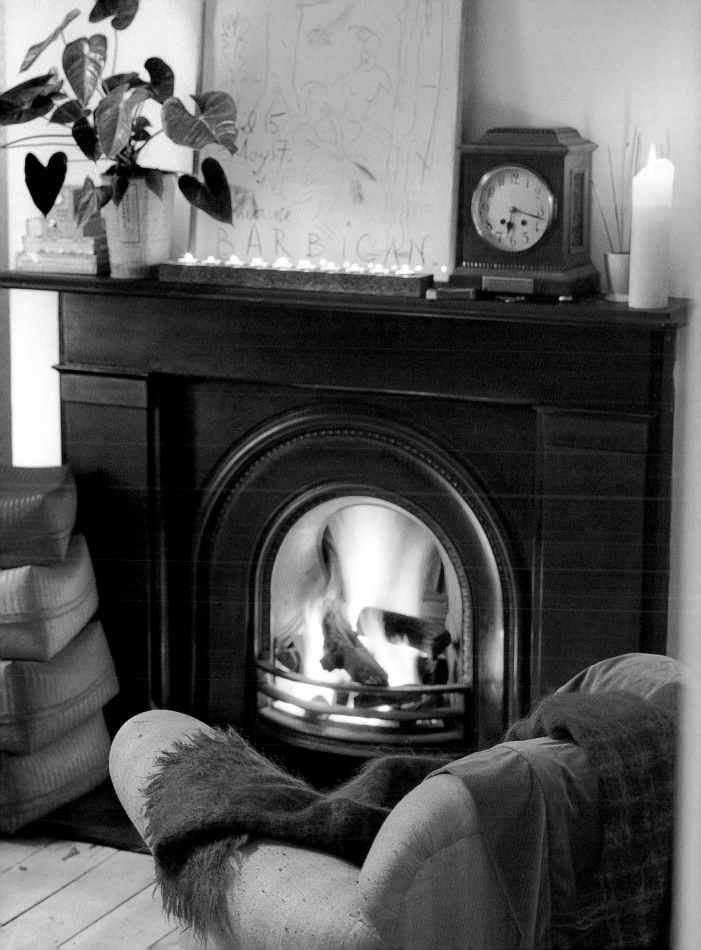

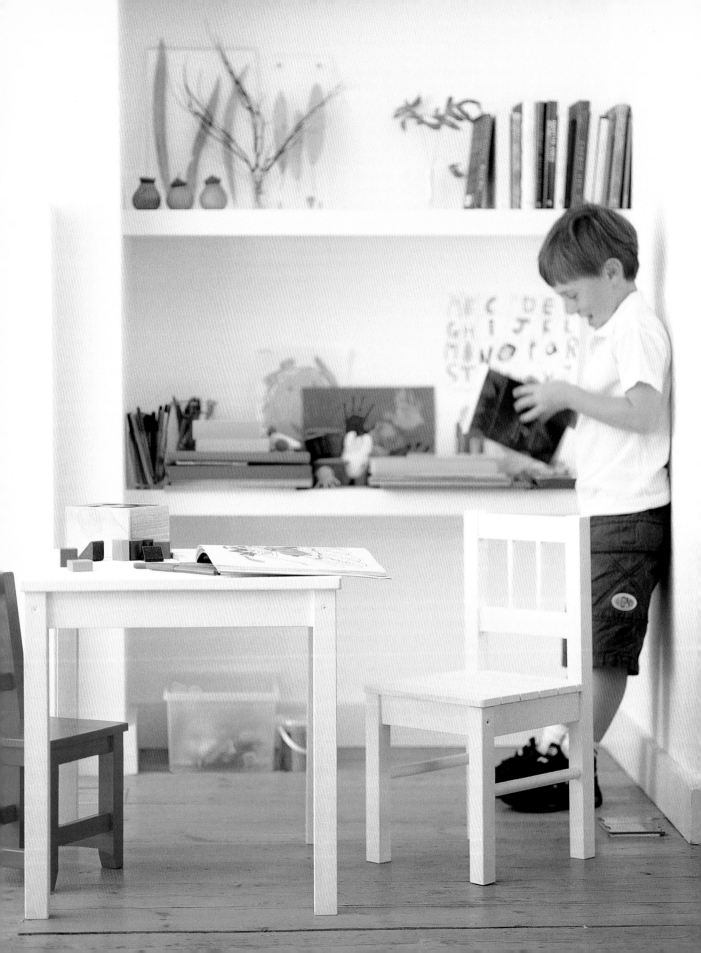

creating personal space for kids

Every parent wants the best for their children. Establishing an environment where children can use their creative and inventive abilities will encourage the belief that they can fulfil all of their goals in life.

Every human has the capacity for genius. It is how this potential is nurtured and encouraged during childhood that determines whether we achieve it. Believe in your children's innate talents and you will instil in them a gift of self-confidence that will enable them to reach their highest potential.

Children learn by example. Your own attitudes and beliefs will be the foundation for their development. So, become a child again when you become a parent. Reawaken the sense of wonder and joy in your attitude towards learning and they will make the association that learning is fun. What better gift can you pass on to your child?

Imagination

Kids need constant stimulation. They need to be kept amused or interested in something most of the time. This means that throughout the house there should be areas for children to be stimulated in order to feel part of the big picture. It is essential that they feel part of the family that they are able to see what goes on. There should also be one space in which they are allowed to be totally themselves (within reason, of course).

Be inventive in their personal space and make it a place where they can express their true creativity. Use uplifting colours to help the process and make the space visually stimulating. Yellow, red and orange are great colours for a playroom to boost energy and create an atmosphere of inspiration.

Independence day

Children need to learn their own way by doing things for themselves. Stocking their play area with creative and interactive toys is the best way to give them the tools they need. Keep a good selection of colourful books, building blocks or toys, pencils, paper, paint, crayons and games.

A great solution for budding artists is to paint a wall in chalkboard paint and let them at it. What a great sense of freedom to be able to draw on the walls! Other ideas for their creative space are to have a table, at the right height, and good lighting and a warm play area on the floor for more active games. Encourage their enthusiasm by always taking the time to praise their efforts. It will make your child want to strive harder and learn more.

Sharing together

Throughout the rest of your house, think about scale. A house must be quite overwhelming through the eyes of a child. As far as they are concerned, there are always interesting things going on above their head, but trying to reach for things ends in disaster. If children want to be involved in your day-to-day activities, find a way of letting them participate on a smaller scale. Have an area in each room where they can play. Whatever you are doing, finding a creative way to get them to participate will make them feel part of the experience.

Remember that home is where your children receive love and security. It needs to be a place where they can grow and flourish and, most importantly, learn. By creating a nurturing personal space for your children, you will help them become inquisitive, independent and self-confident adults who will remember their childhood and home with love and affection.

Every human has the capacity for genius. It is how this potential is nurtured. . .that determines whether we achieve it.

colour your world

Using colour in the home is vitally important as it is the representation of light and, like the amount of light we are exposed to, can dramatically influence how we feel and think. You may notice that you are more likely to feel depressed in the winter months, when the sun sets early and the amount of light is limited. As soon as spring comes around, you get a sudden burst of energy as the days are longer and there is more sunlight. Think of colour in the same way. Give yourself a kick-start by introducing into your home colours that will promote a healthy balance in your life and make you feel happy all year round.

Take a good look around your house or office and see if the colours impact on how you feel. Do you feel energised in certain rooms and contemplative in others? Think about the emotional zones that you need to create within your home to make you feel at your best. You need a space to get a restful night's sleep to enable you to renew your energy. You need to be able to relax and give your mind a rest. You need to be uplifted and inspired. By using the colour palette, we can stimulate these feelings rather than work against them and replenish the vital energy that we need to face each day with a positive attitude.

Why white?

So why do so many of us choose to paint the inside of our homes white? Is it because it's safe to do what everyone else does? Or is it that we just don't know what colour to choose and it's easier to go with white? Although white spaces can look clean and fresh, they really lack warmth and can feel harsh and clinical.

White also shows up any imperfections and, because it is the absence of colour, does not add any energy to the space. All the energy in a stark white room must come from the objects and people in it. It's hard work always having to be the centre of attention, which means you can feel drained when sitting in a completely white room for a period of time.

White works well in an art gallery, where the focus of the room is the art. It also works well in spaces where there are constant crowds of people who bring with them their own 'colour' or energy. If a neutral look is what you are after, take the edge off and add some warmth to the white.

There are a number of nearly white shades that give just a hint of colour, which will change the atmosphere in a room without losing the clarity and cleanliness of pure white. For a more natural base, try off-white or cream, which will add a depth and richness whilst retaining the 'clean' look, and see how different the space feels.

Passionate colours

The fiery, passionate colours, such as red, orange and purple, create an intensity that is not suitable for everyone. My house is predominantly filled with these three colours and always attracts attention. I love the energy and intensity that they emit and I find them all conducive to creativity. On a daily basis, passers-by gather in front of my kitchen window to stare inside at my orange-red walls and hot pink cupboards.

Try these colours as accents before you go all the way. Live with them for a while and see how they make you feel. As they are such dramatic colours, they are more likely to make a great impact in your life or to clash horribly with your home or your favourite possessions. Try them and see. They are not for the weak at heart.

Red

Red is the first colour of the spectrum and has the greatest intensity. It is a colour associated with danger, fire and passion and can be quite aggressive , but it also stimulates your energy levels. For this reason, it is best not to use it in a bedroom or bathroom, where you will want to remain calm and relaxed, but try it in a dining room or kitchen where the intensity will work. If you use it in an area where you entertain frequently you will never have to worry about dull parties.

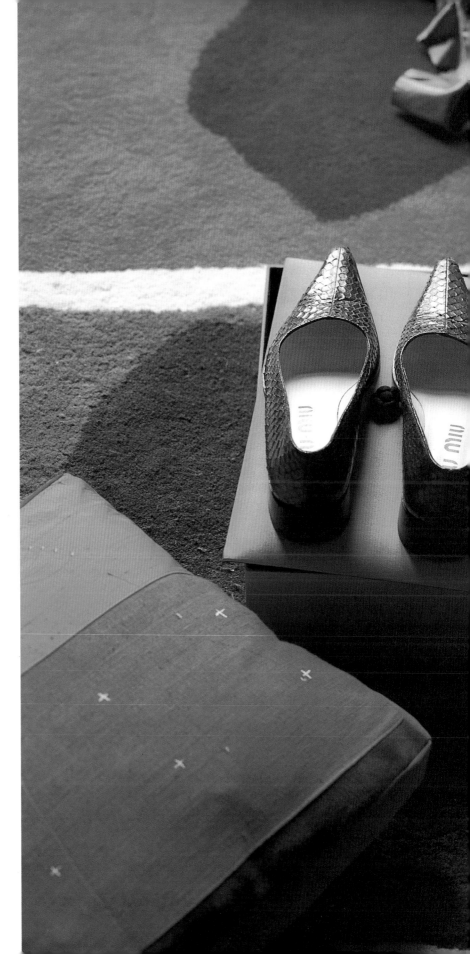

Orange

Orange combines the fire of red with the brown of the earth and is a friendlier, less aggressive colour to live with than bright red. It is vibrant, optimistic and very welcoming, so it's good to use in areas of your home that don't get enough natural sunlight. A very warm colour, it keeps you in an upbeat frame of mind. If bright orange just won't work in your space or will clash dreadfully with your favourite objects, try a softer terracotta tone. Reminiscent of hot Mediterranean holidays, it will give your room a warm richness that will relax and revive you at once.

Purple

Purple is a colour that we associate with religious ritual and royalty. Because of its sacred nature, purple is good in areas of your home where you need a clear head. Use it in your bedroom if you want it to be a place to sit and quietly meditate, and in any rooms that are used for parties or big occasions.

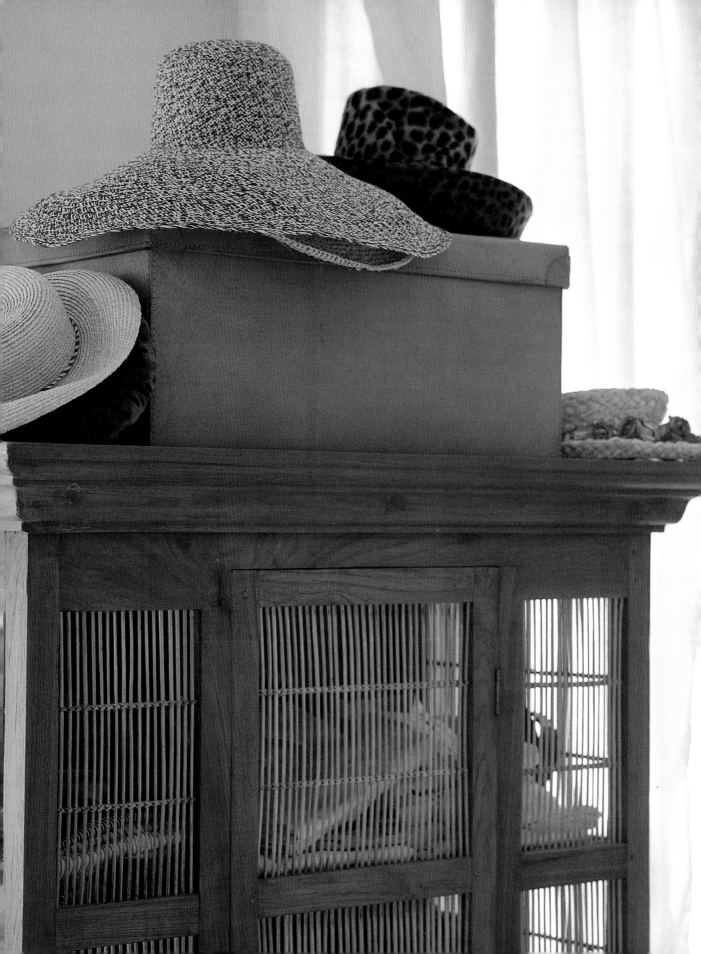

Natural wonders

The colours that we associate with nature have a particularly powerful impact on our mood and can be used throughout our homes to stimulate our senses and bring restorative balance into our lives. There are a variety of tones within each colour, all of which will promote a slightly different response – find the tone that works best for you.

Yellow

Think about the energy and warmth of the sun and you will understand the colour yellow. It is uplifting and focuses your mind. It is cheerful, bright, fresh and stimulating, reminiscent of springtime and new beginnings.

Because of all these connotations, yellow is a great colour to use in your kitchen or dining room, where inspiration and focus are a great way to help start and end the day. The cheerfulness of the colour makes it great for any spaces where people congregate. Try it out in kids' rooms to make their disposition sunnier!

Green

Think about the colour green and what springs to mind is growth, fertility and freshness. It is a very balanced and reassuring colour which can be used anywhere in your home that may require more peace and balance. Because it is associated with abundance and money, it is also considered a lucky colour. It is a good choice for bedrooms or sitting rooms, where you don't need too much stimulation but would like harmony.

Blue

Blue is associated with the sea and sky and represents calmness and tranquillity. Use it in areas where stress or tension has been a problem in the past. It is a very restful colour and is a great choice for a bedroom or bathroom. If, however, you have a tendency to feel blue and have low energy levels, it can add to your woes. You might want to choose a tone that has a higher proportion of red, which will add more energy than a stark, cool blue.

Brown

Brown is the colour of Mother Earth and symbolises stability and strength. If you are constantly up in the air and find it difficult to make decisions, a little touch of brown in a room can bring you back to earth. However, brown can sometimes be seen as depressing, as it also represents the ageing process, so it is probably wise to use it in relatively small doses. As it is a dark colour it can also make a room look much smaller so make sure that you have enough light or space for this not to be a problem!

Grey

Grey is a colour often used as a neutral backdrop in homes and offices. It is a combination of black, which is the absorption of all colours, and white, the absence of colour, and so it is somewhat confused. It can be a soft and subtle colour, but for some it can be depressing as it is reminiscent of stormy, cloudy skies. If you find that you are unsettled in a grey room, this may be the reason.

Colour me happy

Why are we afraid to experiment with colour? A simple pot of paint can transform your room into an emotional haven. It can stimulate your senses and give you energy, or calm the mind and quieten the spirit. All it takes is a little time, a few pots of paint and a brush.

Try a sample wall and live with it for a while. Pay attention to how it makes you feel. If the colour seems too strong, add some white and lighten it up or choose a slightly softer tone. The worst thing that can happen is that you don't like the colour – and all you need do is paint it again. Stretch yourself and take a risk. The results can change your life.

Give yourself a kick-start by introducing into your home colours that will promote a healthy balance . . . and make you feel happy.

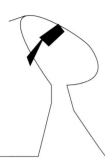

light up your life

When I first moved to England from America, it was in early summer. The weather was in a depression. Day after day, the sky was grey all day long. It went on for months. I was deeply depressed. I had no energy. Each day I walked around my mews house and turned on every light, searching for that brightness that lifts the spirit and lets you know that all is well with the world.

Lighting, either natural or artificial, creates the indefinable character of your home. In my view, it is the most important element of interior design. Lighting gives you the ability to manipulate moods. It can dramatically change your outlook on life. Listen to an artist or photographer describe the quality of light, and it is magical. It is an event. Think about a sunset or the light in the sky before a thunderstorm: it evokes passion. Think of a room lit only by candles: it is charged with emotion. Light streaming through a window inspires dreams.

Get to the source

Artificial light is needed to complement the natural light in our surroundings. Aside from setting the mood we have to see what we're doing. Different areas of the house have different requirements.

Incandescent

Incandescent is the most common type of lighting – the standard bulb used in most lamps and fixtures in your home. Incandescent bulbs are available in different colours and wattages, which will effect their output of light. They use the most amount of electricity.

Fluorescent

Traditionally, fluorescent lighting is thought of as long tubes that give off a raw, blue tone of light and drain away colour. Times have changed. Fluorescent light is now available in warmer tones and traditional light-bulb shapes. It gives off a more even light with little glare and is energy-efficient. The initial cost per bulb is greater but they usually last 10 times longer than incandescent bulbs.

Halogen

Halogen is the closest to the natural, white light of the sun and allows your eyes to see the broadest range of colours. It is for this reason that I always use halogen when I can. Halogen is not without its pitfalls. The

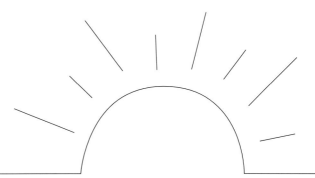

bulbs are very tricky and can burst if you touch them. Once installed, the bulbs get very hot indeed, so they are not ideal for all areas of your house.

Let there be light

There are three different types of lighting in your home. General lighting adds overall light to the room. Task lighting is the light you require to do certain activities – reading, cooking, working, applying make-up, etc. Accent lighting is used to emphasise a design element within a room or highlight a favourite object.

General lighting

The general lighting in your home is usually there when you move in. Recessed ceiling lights, surface-mounted lighting, track lights or a hanging ceiling pendant are the most common. Combined with the natural lighting from your windows, this creates the overall impression of how light your space feels.

Task lighting

Task lighting is the easiest to get right. It is very specific to particular areas of your house and there are lots of choices available. The most common task light is a lamp.

What you want to accomplish is a light source that illuminates the specific area without harshness and glare. Positioning a table lamp also merits consideration. When you are sitting down, the bottom of the lamp shade should be below eye level.

Bathroom lighting is very important to make you look and feel your best. You need a light source by your mirror that provides good, even lighting without shadows. Halogen or a warm fluorescent light around your mirror will make sure that the make-up you apply in the bathroom looks the same in the natural light outdoors.

Accent lighting

Accent lighting highlights a design feature of your home or a favourite object. A light hanging over a painting, lighting inside shelving units or focused on a plant can create drama. Remember that accent lighting requires the object to be lit three times more strongly than the rest of the room for it to stand out from the general light.

Fitting out

There are numerous types of fitting available for all the different kinds of light. Some fittings will work with whichever light source you choose, such as halogen or fluorescent, but many will be designed for a particular source and for a specific use. Check before you buy anything.

Recessed lighting

My preference is always recessed halogen downlighting. It blends into the ceiling and is inconspicuous. The recessed fittings can be stationary, which means that they can only light downwards, or 'eyeball', which means they can rotate through a 45° angle. Halogen provides a natural, warm light.

Recessed halogen lighting can, however, be expensive. It requires ceiling space in which to hide the fixtures and must be installed by an electrician. Recessed lighting should be evenly distributed in the room and should be positioned 60cm–90cm (2–3ft) from the junction with your walls.

Track lighting

Track lighting is much easier to install than recessed lighting and is available for all types of light source – you can also add fittings if necessary. The individual lights can be positioned on the track to illuminate specific areas of your room. Lights are available as spot, which illuminate a small area, or flood, which give a more general wash of light over a greater area. Track lighting can also be used as task lighting to illuminate a specific area, such as kitchen work surfaces.

Ceiling-mounted fixtures

For a more subdued general lighting effect, a single fixture hung from the ceiling in the middle of the room can also provide the general lighting required, although it will probably need to be supplemented by other fixtures. This usually becomes a design feature of the room, as your eye will be attracted to the single source of light. Choose your fitting well and make sure that you clean it regularly.

Wall fixtures and lamps

Wall fixtures, standard lamps that throw light upwards and table lamps can also provide general illumination. Think about how you want your room to feel before deciding on the right option.

Clean up your act

Before you assess how your existing lighting works for you, try a shocking experiment. Dust all the light bulbs, lampshades, and any other fixtures in your house. Look at the difference a good cleaning makes. Replace all the bulbs that don't work. Write down all the different types of bulbs you have in your house and get a supply. There should never be an excuse for a burned-out light bulb.

A ray of light

Armed with the knowledge of the basics, have a good wander through your house over a weekend. Spend time in each room at different times of the day and see how it feels. Jot things down in your notebook. Good lighting should not only make you feel good, but look good.

Make the small changes first. Change a lamp shade and see how it can affect the atmosphere of the space. If your room just seems dull, increase the wattage of your bulbs, if your fixture allows. All lighting comes with recommended wattage instructions, so do ensure that you are not exceeding these. If you want a higher wattage than is recommended for the fixture that you already have, you should buy a new fixture that can take the higher wattage.

Look at your window treatments and how they enhance or restrict the natural lighting available from your windows. Better yet, look at your windows. If they are dirty, they will let in less light. Step by step, make small improvements in each room. Live with them for a while and see how it feels. When you go into a space that you feel really comfortable in, pay attention to the lighting. See what type of lighting has been used to create the mood. It may be possible for you to create the same feeling in your own home.

See how different types of light work with the colours you have chosen for your home. Some types of light may create a glare when bounced off a particular colour or finish on the walls, floors or worktops. Try things out. See how the look and feel of a room can be changed. Let the light shine on.

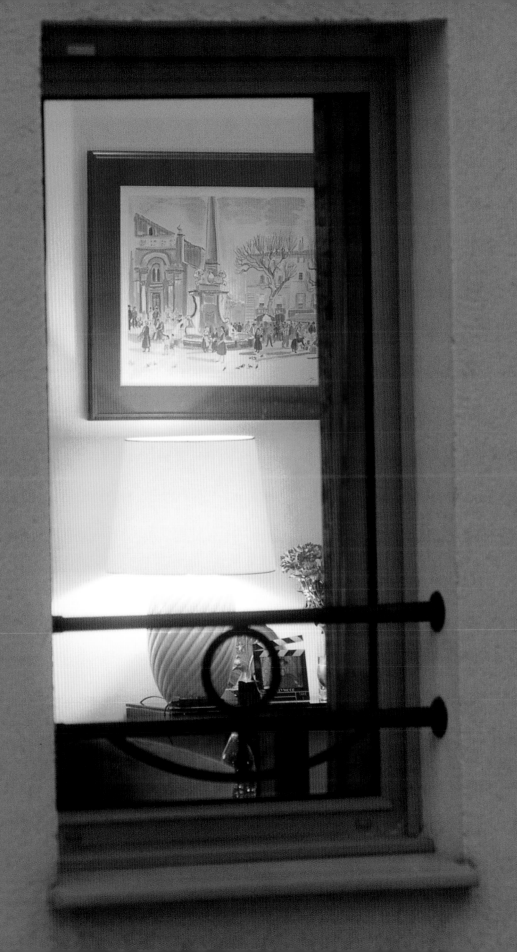

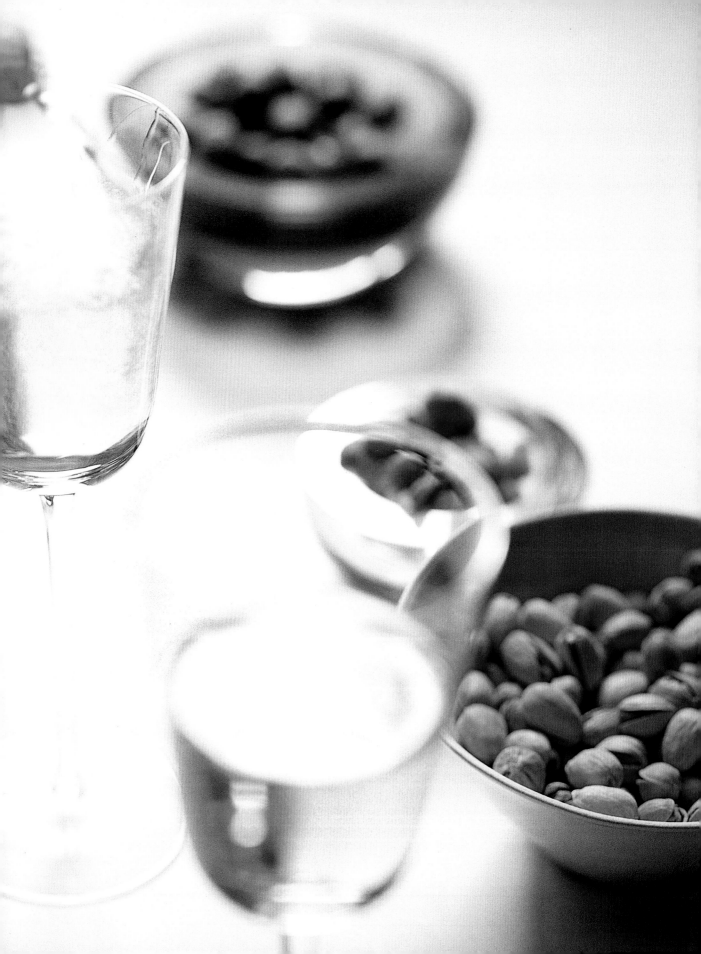

entertaining

"We cherish our friends not for their ability to amuse us, but for ours to amuse them" EVELYN WAUGH

The art of being a great host or hostess is in choosing your companions well, looking after their every need and making it all seem perfectly effortless. An excellent addition to the list, I always think, is never running out of drink!

Entertaining has changed dramatically over the last 20 years. Think about what your parents' dinner parties were like. Formal dining rooms and seven-course dinners have evolved into group gatherings in the kitchen, with a less rigid and much healthier attitude towards food. Meat and two veg are no longer the expected fare. The availability of fresh herbs, ethnic ingredients and inspiring cookery books make imagination the only limitation when organising a dinner party. Have fun with it.

Do as much as possible of the cooking in advance. Make sure that you know what your guests like to eat and, more importantly, if there is anything that they don't or can't eat. Plan a menu and ensure that you have all of the ingredients. There is nothing worse than a panic minutes before your guests arrive. Study the recipes and make sure that everything can fit into the oven for the required cooking times. I remember a very large Thanksgiving turkey and a roasting pan that wouldn't fit into my oven, with 12 guests arriving for dinner – it naturally ended in tears. Don't take anything for granted!

Make it a rule to clean as you go. Try to get all of the preparation dishes washed before the guests arrive. There will be less to do when they leave and you will be thankful to be able to get to bed a bit earlier. Always finish cleaning up before you go to bed: as we all know, dirty dishes are horrible to face in the morning. Share the responsibility with those you live with.

For guests staying overnight for any length of time, make sure that you have stocked the guest room with both the essentials and the pleasures. If you have pets, make sure that your guests know in advance, just in case they have allergies. Give guests a tour of the house and let them know where you keep the coffee, tea and sugar so that they can help themselves if they are the first to get up. Make them comfortable. Be happy to let people into your life.

consuming passions

Cooking stimulates your senses. Close your eyes and conjure up some of your favourite foods. If you try, right now, you can smell the aroma of freshly baked bread, or a chicken roasting in the oven. If you take the time, you can savour the many delicate flavours combined to produce any dish. You can remember occasions when food was the stimulus for great, relaxed gatherings of family and friends. The aroma of certain spices or herbs can often transport you back to a favourite holiday when meals were an adventure. There is no reason for food not to be as exciting once you're back at home.

Cooking is a labour of love. Whether it is as simple as having to provide nutritious meals on a daily basis for your family, or as inspired as spending hours in the kitchen preparing a feast for friends, ensure that your kitchen is well stocked will make the job more pleasurable.

It's a basic fact of life that we all need to eat every day. It can be something you try to get over and done with as quickly as possible or a real pleasure. Why not take the time to enjoy something that you have to do anyway? Make the most of it. Get into the process. Indulge your senses, even if you are making the simplest meal. Use fresh ingredients. Make it look beautiful. Sit at the table. Eat slowly. Appreciate the flavours. Give thanks.

The dinner party

Prepare as much of the food as you can the night before. Some dishes are actually better if prepared in advance, so have a good look through your cookery books and take a little pressure off. Go for the old favourites that you have cooked a number of times and always love. The less you have to do, the easier it is to keep your guests amused!

If you're not confident about your cooking abilities, don't feel guilty about serving prepared food. I won't tell if you don't. Many food retailers and speciality shops have excellent selections, which get better all the time, so if you really don't have the time or the talent, it's as simple as deciding what to buy. Your favourite restaurants may also be able to help, so give them a call.

Your wine selection should enhance the flavours of your meal. There are no rules about red or white, just make sure you get the right body to complement the food.

Most wine merchants are passionate about their wine selections and will gladly advise on the best wine for the meal. Tell them your price range and the dishes you are serving. Do this well in advance so that you can drink the wine at the right temperature.

Indulge your senses, even if you are making the simplest meal. Use fresh ingredients. Make it look beautiful. . . Eat slowly. Appreciate the flavours.

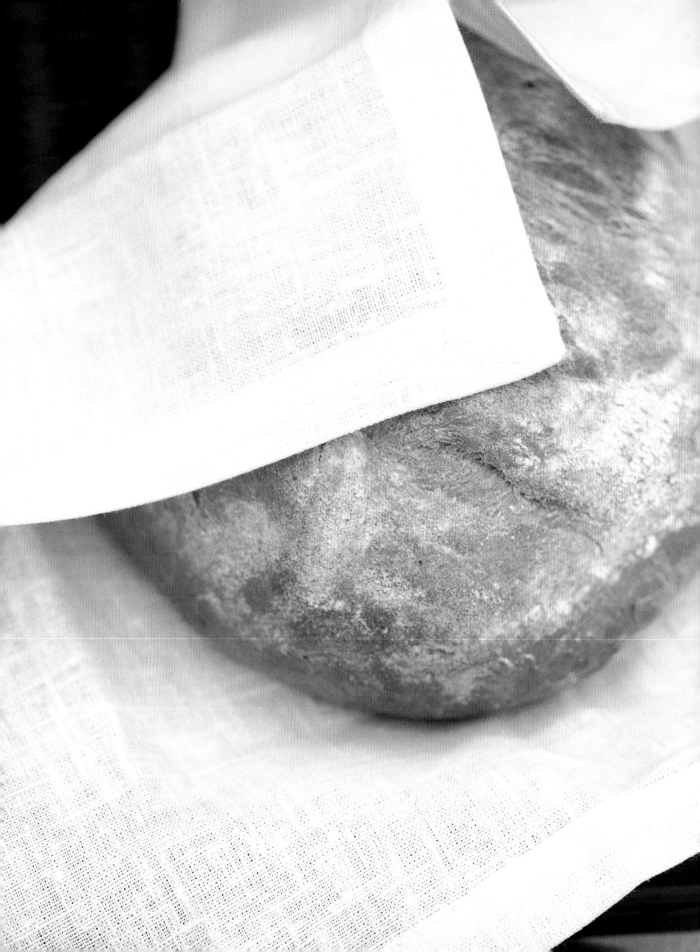

the well-stocked kitchen

Be organised in your kitchen. Save time by keeping your work surfaces clutter-free. If you are going to spend a while cooking, whether just for yourself or for a party of friends, it will make your time in the kitchen much more pleasant if you enjoy your surroundings.

Take a look around your kitchen and make sure that things are stored in the areas you use them. Take stock of your equipment and make sure you have the right tools to help you.

Always buy the best kitchen items you can afford. Look after them and they will last a lifetime. Good pots and pans are essential. The best materials are stainless steel, either with aluminium or copper bases, glass ceramic that are fine to use on the stove, in the oven or microwave, and enamel-coated cast iron.

Make a wish list. Next time you are asked what you would like, have your list to hand. The smallest things can save so much time and can change your attitude to cooking overnight! See how your kitchen stacks up.

Preparation

- Set of 4 nesting mixing bowls

- Good-quality kitchen scales with both grams and ounces

- Large glass measuring jug with liquid measurements

- Set of stainless steel measuring cups

- Set of 4 measuring spoons

- Pestle and Mortar

- Good-quality garlic press

- Vegetable peeler with flexible blade

- Good quality salt and pepper mills

- Flexible rubber spatula

- 2 stainless steel whisks

- 3 wooden spoons

- Heavy-duty can opener

- Heavy-duty bottle opener

- Large stainless steel colander

- Stainless steel flour sifter

- Kitchen tongs

- Long-handled slotted spoon

- Bulb baster

- Meat thermometer

- Citrus zester

- Fruit corer

- Kitchen timer

- Soup ladle

- 4-sided metal grater

- Butcher-block chopping board

- Kitchen string

- Pastry brush

- Kitchen shears

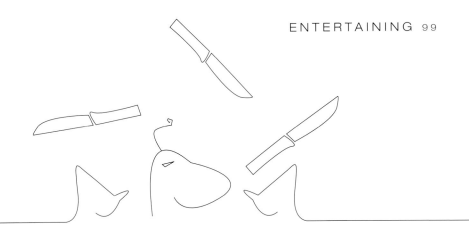

The cutting edge

Have a good selection of knives to hand – make sure that they are stored properly and kept sharpened.

- 2 paring knives – 10cm/4in blade

- Cooks knife – 15cm/6in blade

- Chef's knife – 20cm/8in blade

- Carving knife – 25cm/10in blade

- Bread knife – serrated blade

- Sharpening steel

Kitchen aids

- Heavy-duty food processor

- Toaster

- Electric hand-held mixer

- Kettle

- Coffee pot

- Baking trays

- Ovenproof 23cm/9in glass pie dish

- Baking sheet – 46 x 30 x 2.5cm (18 x 12 x 1in)

- Springform cake tin – 23cm/9in

- Loaf tin – 23 x 13 x 7.5cm (9 x 5 x 3in)

- 2 round cake tins – 23cm/9in

- Rolling pin

- Wire rack

- Muffin or Yorkshire pudding tin

Cooking

Saucepans

You will need three sizes – 1, 2 and 3 litres (1¾, 3½ and 5¼ pints) – all with tight-fitting lids. Ideally they should all be between 7.5cm/3in and 10cm/4in deep. Ovenproof handles make them even more versatile.

Pots

You will need three sizes – 2.5, 5 and 8 litres (4½, 9 and 14¼ pints) – all with tight-fitting lids. The largest pot is great for making soups and stocks.

Frying pans

You will need two – 20cm/8in and 25cm/10in – with oven-proof handles. Ideally, one should be coated with a non-stick surface.

Casseroles

Two dishes are ideal – a 3 litre/5 pints casserole with a lid and another of the same size that can go in the microwave.

Roasting tins

Check the dimensions of your oven to make sure of the size before you buy your tins. An ideal sized roasting tin just fits whatever you are roasting. I have two – 38 x 30 x 8cm (15 x 12 x 3in) for large roasts and a smaller one 33 x 20 x 8cm (13 x 8 x 3in) for joints and smaller roasts.

Folding roasting rack

Stainless steel folding rack that can fit in either roasting tin.

Vegetable steamer

Look for one that is adjustable and fits all sizes of pot.

stocking the larder

You only have to do this once, so even if it takes a few hours to get right, it will save lots of time in the long run. Make a list of all the different food items you keep in your house. On a separate sheet of paper, think about how your supermarket is laid out, and list your items according to the aisle you find them in. It's a great way to test your memory and see how much attention you really pay to your chores.

Photocopy the list to become your weekly shopping list. Before you go to the shops, make sure that you have enough of all your staples to get you through the week. If not, indicate what you need on the list. Check any recipes you are planning for the week that may require special ingredients. Add them to the list. I find it can save me 15–20 minutes each shop. More time to eat!

Organise your food cupboards by category, so that you and all members of the family know where things live. There will be no excuses for not putting away the shopping and you'll always know your stock levels.

These are the cooking ingredients I use most often and always keep to hand. Add or subtract your essentials and start your list.

Beverages
• Coffee – instant, espresso, ground
• Tea – a selection of traditional and
  herbal for all tastes
• Fruit juice or cordial

Baking essentials
• Baking powder
• Bicarbonate of soda
• Baking chocolate – plain
  drops, unsweetened squares
• Cornflour
• Dried fruits – raisins, sultanas,
  apricots, cherries
• Flour – choose the types that
  you use most often
• Extracts – vanilla, almond and any
  others that you use regularly
• Gelatin
• Nuts – almonds,
  pecans, walnuts, hazlenuts
• Sugars – castor, granulated, icing

Condiments
• Capers
• Chutney
• Fruit jams and marmalades
• Horseradish
• Ketchup
• Mustards – a variety is nice.
  Dijon, whole-grain and English
• Olives – green, whole black,
  pitted black
• Oil – vegetable, extra virgin olive,
  sesame, walnut
• Mayonnaise (or salad cream)
• Pickles
• Preserves
• Soy sauce/Teriyaki
• Tabasco sauce
• Vinegar – malt, balsamic, white wine,
  red wine, cider, raspberry
• Worcestershire Sauce

Herbs and spices
• Allspice
• Basil
• Bay leaves
• Cardamom
• Chilli powder
• Cinnamon, ground and stick
• Cloves
• Cumin, ground and seeds
• Curry powder
• Dill
• Fennel seeds
• Ginger, ground
• Mint
• Nutmeg, whole and ground
• Oregano
• Paprika
• Pepper, whole black, ground black
  and white, red chilli flakes
• Rosemary
• Sage
• Salt – table, coarse
• Sesame seeds
• Tarragon
• Thyme

Starch
• Pasta – spaghetti, macaroni, linguine,
  fettuccine, penne
• Rice – basmati, long-grain, brown,
  wild, arborio

Essential mixers
• Stock cubes and gravy granules
• Tinned soups for quick sauces
• Tomatoes – tinned whole plum,
  concentrate, purée, sun-dried in oil

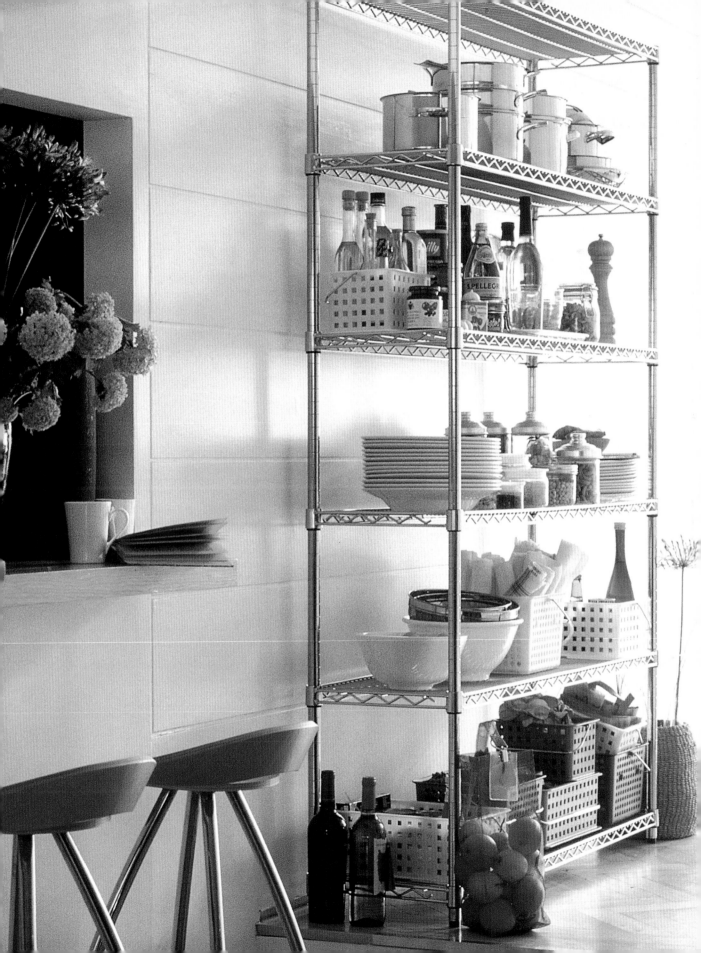

painless party preparations

Parties are a perfect way to thank all your family and friends who do so much to enrich your life. It's a way to say how much you appreciate them being around. Make it a time to enjoy beautiful and delicious food and stimulating conversation. Laugh a lot. Listen to great music. Catch up. Slow down. Really listen to what people are saying. Dance in the kitchen. Take off your watch. Let the good times roll.

Make the time to celebrate. It doesn't have to be a life event. Be spontaneous. Get inspired. The first sight of a spring flower, the middle of the week, vegetables from your garden, or bumping into a friend is reason enough to get connected.

Become one with your kitchen. Enjoy the process. Dance when you cook. Give it all your energy. Make it a labour of love.

Celebration

Every now and then, have a big party, just for the fun of it. Plan every little detail. Start with the guest list. Think about the people that you want to invite. Mix and match people with different points of view. Invite people who don't know each other, along with some that do. Make the group interesting. Let the sparks fly.

Pick a date enough in advance that all of your guests are likely to be available. Send out invitations to set the tone for the evening. Be creative. Make it personal. I had a dinner party at my house for 40 people, where everyone had to wear their favourite pair of shoes. I photographed everyone's feet during the course of the evening and used the photographs in my shop window. It was a giggle.

Have fun. Make sure people know when they are expected. Be specific. Drinks at 7.00pm – Dinner at 8.00pm will get them there before dinner goes cold. Get dressed up. Put on the dog. Know who is coming. Give directions. If you haven't heard from someone, call them. Plan ahead.

Plan a menu

Go through your favourite cookery books and decide on the menu. Make things that you really love to eat, keeping special dietary restrictions of your guests in mind. Don't forget to ask them. Use whatever is in season. Avoid stress in the kitchen by keeping it simple. Don't choose things that require complicated last-minute preparations.

Combine great, fresh flavours with interesting textures during all courses of the meal. Think about how things will look as well as taste, mixing colours as well as flavours. Balance the courses. A creamy dish should be followed by something with bite and texture. A highly seasoned or rich main course should be followed by a lighter, more delicate dessert.

Prepare the way

Do as much of the shopping as you can days ahead. Leave nothing to chance. If you forget something you will have plenty of time to get it. Don't panic.

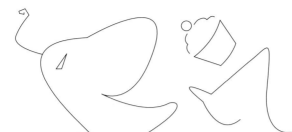

Buy the flowers and let them open. Wash your table linen and make sure you iron it. Polish the silver. Clean the glasses. Buy your wine and let it chill if necessary. Put your candles in the freezer to help them burn longer. Think about how you want your table to look. Think about where you want people to sit. Be eclectic. Mix and match friends, china and glasses. Don't be afraid to let your personality shine through.

Set the table the night before. Forks on the left. Knives and spoons on the right. Pudding cutlery above. Keep them in the order of how you use them. Glasses should go on the right hand side at the top of the plates. Water is first. White wine second. Red wine third. Bread plates go on the left. Be prepared. Know the marching order.

Cook up a storm

Enjoy your time in the kitchen. Put on your apron. Turn up the music. Take your time. Mark the pages of your cookery books and complete stages of the recipes one at a time. Cook as much as you can a day or two in advance. Keep a list of how long things need to be reheated for so you know when to pop things in the oven when the day arrives. Select the serving dishes. Go with the flow.

On the day of the party, go shopping as early as you can for the last-minute necessities. Buy the ingredients for a couple of different cocktails. Prepare these in advance. Clean as you go. Put any dirty dishes through the wash and tidy them away before the guests arrive.

Plan to have at least 45 minutes for yourself before the evening begins. Have a cocktail. Chill out. Put on the music. Check your table. Fill the water glasses with ice-cool mineral water.

Have fun

Light the candles. Greet your guests at the door and offer them a cocktail. Have fresh juice for those who don't drink or are driving. Shake and mingle.

Enjoy your friends. Make introductions and let everyone get to know each other before dinner begins. Cocktails should last no longer than an hour. Slip away to check on progress in the kitchen and get everyone seated as soon as the serving dishes have been placed on the table.

Enlist a friend or partner to help in the serving and clearing. Serve from the left. Clear from the right. Pop the dishes into the dishwasher as you go and things won't overwhelm you when everyone's gone. Clear what is not needed on the table before the last course so that everyone can enjoy the dessert. Refresh the wine.

Coffee, tea and liqueurs can be served anywhere in the house. Unless people are extremely comfortable where they are, move to another room. Gain a different perspective. Have decaffeinated coffee and a selection of teas ready for those who need them. Clear away the cups and glasses. Turn the music up. Dance the night away.

tried and tested recipes

nibbles and starters

Cheese and Onion Spread

Everyone will want this recipe!

SERVES: 8 AS NIBBLES
PREPARATION TIME: 10 MINUTES
COOKING TIME: 45 MINUTES
butter, for the baking dish
1 large sweet (or white) onion
350g/12oz Gruyère
    or Emmenthal cheese
2 tbsp mayonnaise
salt and pepper
crusty French bread or savoury
    biscuits, to serve

1 Preheat the oven to 190°C/375°F/
gas 5 and butter a 26cm/10½in,
round baking dish.
2 Chop the onion into medium-size
dice. Shred the cheese with a grater.
3 In a mixing bowl, mix the two
together and add just enough
mayonnaise to bind them. Season to
taste with salt and pepper and pour
the mixture into a dish.
4 Bake for 45 minutes.

Serve warm with crusty French
bread or savoury biscuits.

WINE TIP: Try an unoaked New
World Chardonnay.

Narsai David's Caponata

*This recipe takes a bit more
preparation time and is even better
if made the night before. Remove
the caponata from the refrigerator
and serve at room temperature as
a starter, or use it as a sauce for a
hearty pasta main course.*

SERVES: 8
PREPARATION TIME: 45 MINUTES
2 large onions
2 red peppers, de-seeded
2 celery sticks
1 medium aubergine
5 tbsp extra virgin olive oil
two 400g/14oz tins plum tomatoes
125g/4½oz sultanas
75g/2¾oz toasted pine nuts
55g/1¾oz capers, drained
75g/2¾oz green olives, chopped
75g/2¾oz Mediterranean black
    olives, chopped
2tbsp white wine vinegar
crusty French bread to serve

1 Chop the onions, peppers,
celery and aubergine into medium-
size pieces.
2 Sauté the aubergine pieces in 2
tablespoons of the olive oil until
brown and tender. Using a slotted
spoon, remove to a large mixing
bowl.
3 In the same pan, sauté the onions,
peppers and celery, adding more oil
as needed.
4 Add the tomatoes, with juice, and
sultanas and simmer for 5 minutes,
scraping all the brown bits up from
the pan.
5 Pour the contents of the pan over
the aubergine. Add the remaining
ingredients, stir to mix well and leave
to stand for 2–3 hours at room
temperature or refrigerate overnight.

Serve at room temperature, with
crusty French bread as a nibble or
over penne or rigatoni.

WINE TIP: Try an Italian red wine
made from Barbera or Sangiovese
grapes.

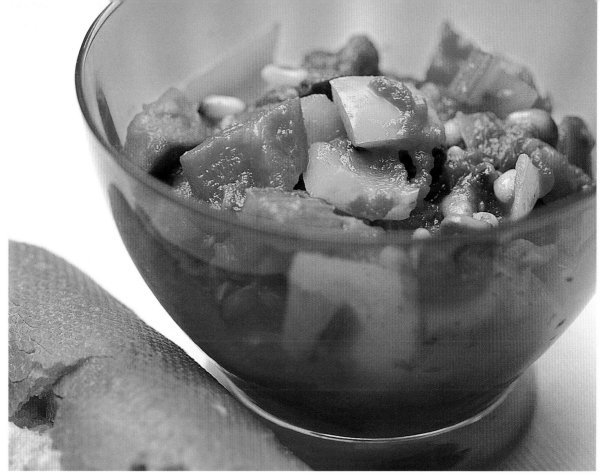

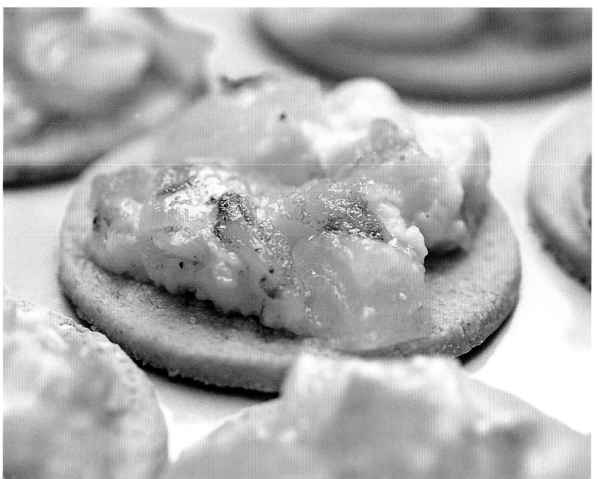

salads and dressings

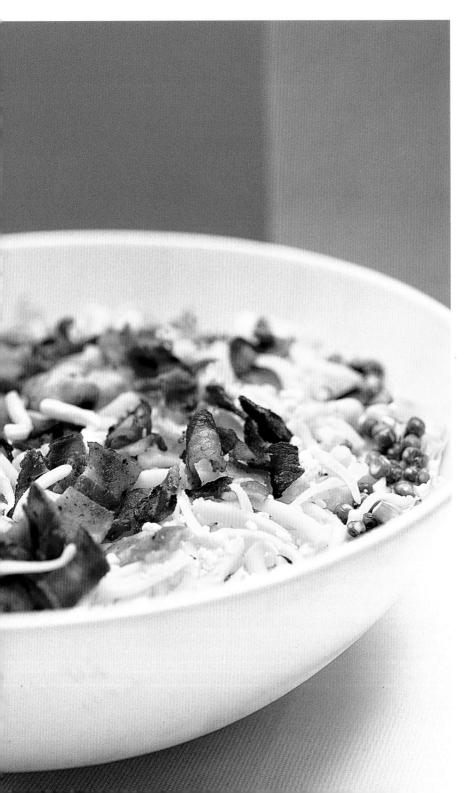

Overnight Lettuce Salad

I have been making this recipe for 20 years. It is a family favourite and, although it may sound strange, it is delicious.

SERVES: 8–10

PREPARATION TIME: 30 MINUTES, PLUS OVERNIGHT STANDING

1 large head of crisp lettuce (preferably iceberg), chopped
2 bunches of spring onions, chopped (using the bulb and 10cm/4in of the greens)
600g/1lb 5oz mayonnaise
150g/5oz sugar
675g/1½lb frozen peas
450g/1lb mild Cheddar cheese, grated
250g/9oz slices of smoked bacon, grilled and cut into small pieces

1 This salad is made in layers. Put the lettuce in a large bowl, then scatter the onions on top.
2 Mix together the mayonnaise and sugar, beating well. Spoon this on top of the lettuce and onions.
3 Add layers of frozen peas, grated cheese and finally the bacon.

Let it sit overnight in a refrigerator before serving.

WINE TIP: Try a Californian Chardonnay or a young Cabernet Sauvignon with this dish.

The Best Vinaigrette Ever

SERVES: 10
PREPARATION TIME: 10 MINUTES
4 tbsp red wine vinegar
2 egg yolks
salt and pepper
4 tbsp Dijon mustard
2 garlic cloves, crushed or finely
   chopped
1 shallot, finely chopped
chopped parsley (amount equal to
   the chopped shallot)
500ml/18fl oz vegetable oil (canola,
   or rapeseed, oil is best for this)

1 Add the vinegar to the egg yolks.
Sprinkle with salt and pepper and
leave to stand for 2–3 minutes.
2 Add the mustard, garlic, shallot
and parsley, and beat on low mixer
speed for 2–3 minutes or hand
whisk. With the machine still running,
add the oil in a slow stream, gradually
increasing the mixer speed, and beat
until it has the desired consistency.

This is great served over greens or
baby lettuces.

WINE TIP: Try a young Loire
wine – Sancerre or Pouilly Fumé –
or a New Zealand Sauvignon.

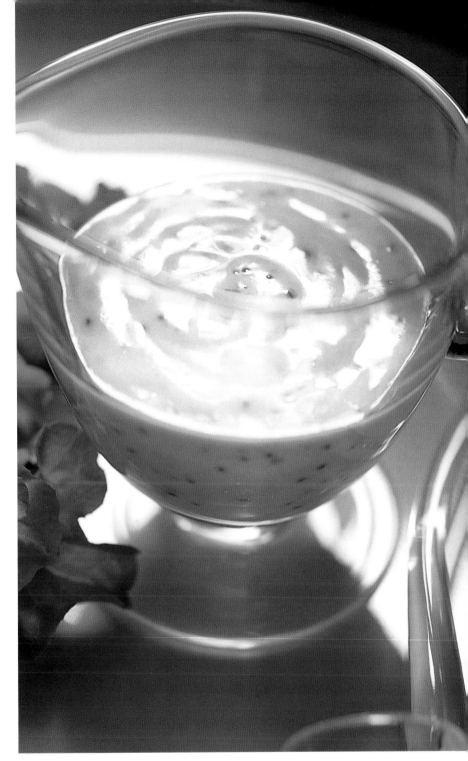

main courses

Fillet of Beef Wrapped in Herbs

This is one my favourite recipes from The Silver Palette Cookbook. *It is a very simple dish to prepare and is great for a large crowd. Go to a good butcher and ask them to wrap the fillet in beef fat, tied loosely. Make sure they weigh it before they put the fat on! Prepare the beef the night before and all you have to do is pop it into the oven when the crowd arrives.*

SERVES: 8–10
PREPARATION TIME: 15 MINUTES
COOKING TIME: 45 MINUTES
1 fillet of beef, about 1.8kg/4lb
bunch fresh rosemary
bunch fresh thyme
bunch fresh oregano
2 garlic cloves, slivered
salt and pepper

1 Preheat the oven to 220°C/425°F/gas 7.
2 Remove the fat from the fillet and place the herbs lengthwise all around the meat. Put the fat around the herbs and meat and tie the string snugly.
3 Cut deep slits through the fat into the meat and insert the slivered garlic firmly into the meat. Sprinkle generously with salt and freshly ground pepper.

4 Place the fillet in a roasting tin just large enough to hold it with ease. Bake for 10 minutes on the high heat, then reduce the oven setting to 180°C/350°F/gas 4 and cook for 25 minutes more for rare meat or 35 minutes for medium.
5 Remove the roast from the oven and let it rest in a warm place for 10 minutes. Remove the fat and herbs and slice the beef as you prefer.

This is best served with new potatoes and a green salad. Use the herb and garlic rich drippings in the tin to make a tasty accompanying gravy. Skim off the layer of fat on the top, add gravy granules and heat slowly on the hob.

WINE TIP: Try a full-bodied red wine such as a young red Bordeaux, Châteauneuf du Pape, Sonoma County Zinfandel or Southern Australian Shiraz.

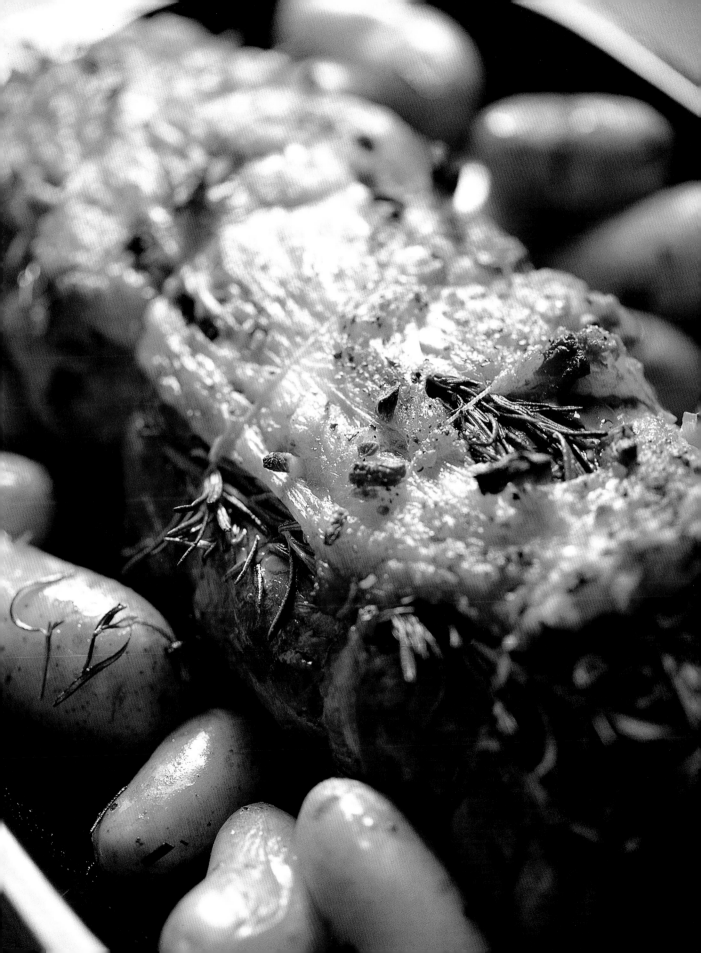

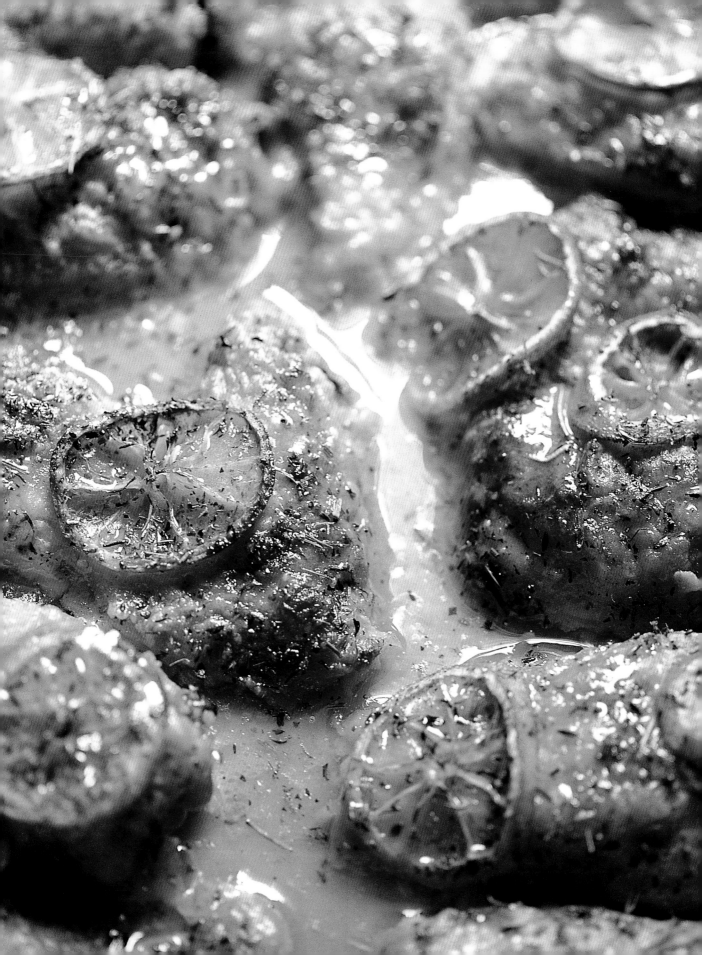

Lemon Chicken

This dish is wonderful served at any temperature, which makes it ideal for a picnic. It's great for a crowd – just double the recipe. It is best made the night before, allowing the chicken to marinate in the lemon.

SERVES: 8–10
PREPARATION TIME: 15 MINUTES
COOKING TIME: 60–65 MINUTES, INCLUDING
  OVERNIGHT STANDING TIME

11 lemons
Two 1kg/2¼lb chickens, quartered
250g/9oz flour
1 tsp sweet paprika
salt and pepper
2 tsp light brown sugar
250ml/9fl oz chicken stock
1 tsp herbes de Provence

1 Squeeze 10 of the lemons and retain the juice.
2 Place the chicken pieces in a shallow dish and pour the lemon juice over them. Leave to marinate overnight, or for as long as possible, turning the pieces occasionally.
3 When ready to cook, preheat the oven to 190°C/375°F/gas 5.
4 In a mixing bowl, combine together the flour, paprika, salt and pepper to taste.
5 Remove the pieces of marinated chicken from their dish, reserving the lemon juice for later, and toss them in the flour mixture. I always find the easiest way to get an even coating of flour is to place the flour mixture in a plastic bag, drop the chicken pieces into it and shake it around until all the pieces are coated.
6 When evenly coated, place the chicken pieces skin-side up in a shallow baking tin and cook in the preheated oven for 40 minutes.
7 While the chicken is cooking, thinly slice the last lemon. Whisk together the reserved lemon juice, brown sugar and chicken stock and then add the lemon slices.
8 After the chicken has been cooking for 40 minutes, pour the lemon mixture over it and sprinkle with the herbs. Cook for a further 20–25 minutes.

If eating cold, serve with cold wild rice salad. If eating hot, serve with warm wild rice and a green salad.

WINE TIP: Try a fruity red Sancerre.

Crab Quiche

This is so quick and easy to prepare and is always a winner!

SERVES: 4–6 PER QUICHE
PREPARATION TIME: 10 MINUTES
   (NOT INCLUDING PIE CRUST)
COOKING TIME: 35 MINUTES
2 ready-made pie shells (better yet,
   use the pie crust recipe, right)
450g/1lb crab meat
2 eggs
250ml/9fl oz mayonnaise
125ml/4fl oz milk
4 tbsp flour
bunch spring onions, green parts
   included, chopped
450g/1lb Gruyère cheese, shredded
paprika
salt and pepper

1 Preheat the oven to 180°C/350°F/ gas 4. Prepare pie shells (or fresh pastry). Check the crabmeat for any shell fragments.
2 Beat the eggs in a small bowl and add the mayonnaise, milk and flour. Pour into a larger bowl, add the crab meat, spring onions and cheese. Season with salt and pepper and mix.
3 Divide the crab mixture evenly between the two pie shells and spread evenly. Sprinkle lightly with paprika. Bake for 35 minutes.

Serve with green salad with a home-made vinaigrette dressing (see p. 107).

WINE TIP: Try a fresh Sauvignon Blanc or a soft Chardonnay.

Pie Crust

These quantities are enough for one pie with a top and bottom layer or two shells.

PREPARATION TIME: 15 MINUTES
375g/13oz bleached plain flour
1 tsp salt
115g/4oz cold butter, cut into pieces
6 tbsp cold solid vegetable shortening
   (such as Trex)
5–6 tbsp iced water

1 Combine the flour and salt in a mixing bowl. Add the butter and shortening and working quickly, using a pastry blender, two knives or your fingertips, cut in the ingredients until the mixture resembles coarse crumbs.
2 Sprinkle the iced water over the mixture a tablespoon at a time, and toss the dough after each addition. When you can gather the dough into a ball, you have added enough water.
3 Transfer the dough onto a cool, lightly floured surface and, taking about ½ cup at a time, use the heel of your hand to smear the dough away from you, Repeat until all the dough has been blended.
4 Gather the dough into a ball and divide it in half. Flatten slightly, wrap each section in cling-film and chill in a refrigerator for 30 minutes. It could also be frozen at this stage for later use.
5 Roll the chilled dough out on a lightly floured surface and then use to line your pie dish.

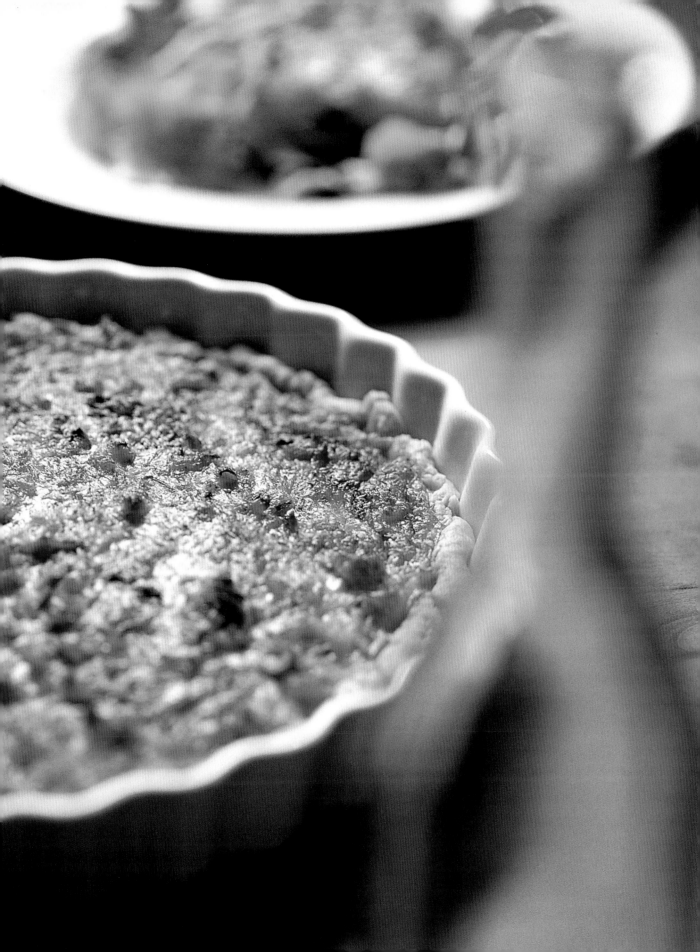

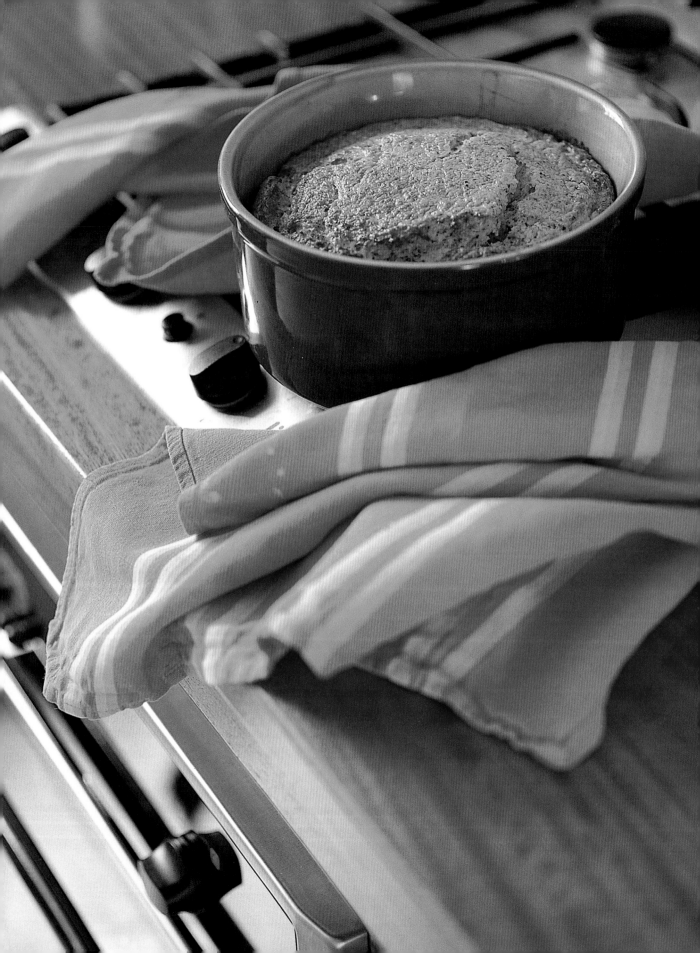

Vegetable Soufflé

This can be used as a starter or a main course. As with all soufflés, it should be served straight from the oven, so make sure that your guests are seated before you take it out.

SERVES: 6
PREPARATION TIME: 10 MINUTES
COOKING TIME: 1 HOUR
3 tbsp butter
3 tbsp flour
250ml/9fl oz milk
3 eggs
6 spring onions, chopped
350g/12oz any uncooked vegetable
   (broccoli, asparagus or corn)
salt and pepper

1 Preheat the oven to 180°C/350°F/ gas 4.
2 In a medium-sized saucepan, melt the butter over a medium heat. Add the flour and stir into the butter for 2–3 minutes. Slowly add the milk and stir until very thick and smooth. Pour into a food processor fitted with a steel blade.
3 Add the eggs, onions, vegetables, salt and pepper and process in short bursts until the mixture is well combined but with some texture remaining.
4 Pour the mixture into an ungreased 1 litre/1¾ pint soufflé or Pyrex dish. Bake for 1 hour until risen.

Serve immediately with green salad.

WINE TIP: Try an unoaked Chardonnay.

Chilled Lebanese Soup

My friend Tessa is a most inspired cook – this recipe is hers. It has a stunning combination of flavours and is so simple to prepare. Make one day before you plan to serve it. Thank you, Tessa!

SERVES: 4 AS A MAIN OR 6 AS A STARTER
PREPARATION TIME: 10 MINUTES, PLUS
   24 HOURS' STANDING TIME
400ml/14fl oz Greek yoghurt
250ml/9fl oz single cream
1 cucumber, cut in half lengthways,
   de-seeded, with skin on
4 gherkins, chopped
3 tbsp capers
125g/4½oz tiger prawns
2 tbsp chopped fresh tarragon
1 lemon
1 bunch mint

1 In a large bowl, mix together the Greek yoghurt and single cream.
2 Grate the cucumber into the same bowl. Add the chopped gherkins, capers, prawns and tarragon. Stir to mix well.
3 Cover the bowl and place it in a refrigerator for 24 hours.
4 To serve, pour the chilled soup into bowls, squeeze over a little lemon juice and sprinkle with chopped mint.

Serve with pitta bread as a starter, or with crusty French bread as a main course. Try scooping out the inside of a rustic loaf and filling it with the soup. Use the remaining bread to dunk.

WINE TIP: Try a Sauvignon Blanc.

desserts

Pecan Puffs

MAKES 36

PREPARATION TIME: 20 MINUTES

COOKING TIME: 30 MINUTES

225g/8oz butter, plus extra for the
 baking sheet
15g/½oz castor sugar
1 tsp good-quality vanilla extract
100g/3½oz whole pecans, ground
140g/4½oz sifted cake flour
icing sugar, to dust
good-quality vanilla ice cream, to
 serve (optional)

1 Preheat the oven to 150°C/300°F/
gas 2 and butter a baking sheet.
2 Beat the butter until soft. Add the
sugar and blend until creamy. Add
the vanilla, then stir in the pecans
and flour.
3 Form this dough into about 36
small balls.
4 Place the balls on the prepared
baking sheet, with at least ½cm gap
between each, and bake for about
30 minutes. Take from the oven and,
while they are still hot, coat them in
the icing sugar.

I always serve these biscuits with a
good-quality vanilla ice cream.

WINE TIP FOR DESSERTS: Try a
sweet dessert wine, such as a good
Italian Moscato or a late harvest
Orange Muscat from Australia.

Summer Fruit Cake

SERVES: 10

PREPARATION TIME: 10 MINUTES

COOKING TIME: 1 HOUR

115g/4oz melted butter, plus extra
 for the tin
150g/5oz flour, plus extra for the tin
225g/8oz whole, uncooked berries
 (raspberries and blueberries)
30–60g/1–2oz pecans, chopped
350g/12oz sugar
2 eggs
icing sugar, to dust
slightly sweetened whipped cream,
 to serve

1 Preheat the oven to 160°C/325°F/
gas 3. Grease and flour a 23cm/9in
springform cake tin.
2 Pick through the berries and
remove any stems or leaves.
3 Pour the berries into the tin, then
sprinkle the pecans and a third of
the sugar over them.
4 In a medium bowl, mix together
the eggs, flour, melted butter and
the rest of the sugar. Pour this
mixture over the berries. Note ,the
batter will be thick – pour it slowly
over all the berries.
5 Bake for 1 hour in preheated oven.
6 Turn out upside down on a plate
and sprinkle with icing sugar.

Serve with slightly sweetened
whipped cream.

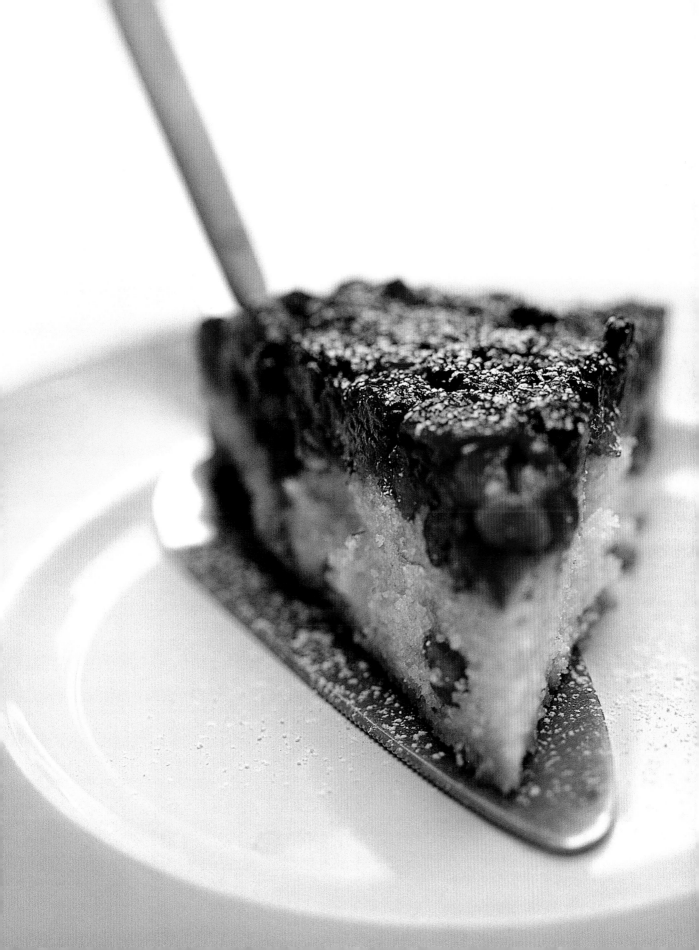

which wine

Like a passionate cook, an ardent wine connoisseur indulges their senses. First they look at the colour and then they smell the aromas wafting from the glass. They choose the best vessel to enhance the flavours. They breathe in while they take the first sip so that the aroma and flavour combine and enhance each other. They close their eyes and focus on the complex tastes. They can identify, in a sip, a hint of elderflower, freshly mown grass, musky earth or the taste of a peach. They take the time to slowly understand the character and age of what they are drinking. They can feel the acidity or the sweetness on their tongue. They enjoy the complete experience.

Take the time to choose the perfect wines to enhance the flavours of all the dishes on your menu. Sample a variety. Buy a wine book and learn about the different types of grape and their characteristics. Really taste and appreciate. Try to detect the separate flavours in each wine. Savour the moment. Put your feet up. Kick back. Pour yourself a big glass. See. Smell. Taste. Smile.

Be informed. Ask for help at your local wine merchant. Tell them what kind of meal you are preparing and ask for their recommendations. Listen to their descriptions of different wines.

With over 10,000 grape varieties and a diverse group of wine-growing countries, there are now more choices available than ever. I've asked wine expert Amanda Skinner, from John Armit Wines in London, to give a description of some of the noble grape varieties and the types of food that each complements.

Sauvignon Blanc

The classic aromas of wines made from Sauvignon Blanc grapes include freshly mown hay, gooseberry, herbs, elderflowers, citrus fruit and peel – all enticing and vibrant noses. The best Sauvignons tend to be fresh and clean on the palate, with relatively high levels of acidity, and intense but not cloying or overpowering flavours. Most are drinkable with or without food.

They are a very good partner for shellfish, fish, spiced dishes – particularly Thai spices – and salads incorporating the 'difficult' ingredients of tomato, peppers and asparagus. The acidity combines with cheeses very successfully, particularly mild creamy cheeses and goat's cheese. Sauvignon is also a good grape variety to serve with plainly cooked chicken and pork.

Chardonnay

While Sauvignon Blanc produces its best wines in cooler climates, Chardonnay is a grape that travels well, and because it flourishes in many different soils and climates, its characteristics are equally varied. Burgundy is undoubtedly the home of the greatest wines made from the Chardonnay grape and the aromas you would expect to associate with these wines include butter, nuts, honey and beeswax.

These are really full-bodied, 'food' wines that perfectly complement many seafood dishes such as lobster, wild salmon, fleshy white fish and scallops, particularly if served with rich sauces. Chardonnays from around the world can be overpoweringly oaky at their worst, but at their best they are elegant and complex. They share many characteristics with Burgundy, but have a slightly more tropical scent.

Pinot Noir

This grape is a bad traveller and is really most successful at home in Burgundy. It is the grape of the great wines of Nuits St Georges, Gevrey Chambertin, Savigny les Beaune, Volnay and many more.

It prefers a cool climate and is difficult to grow as the vine is vulnerable to rot and disease. In too warm an environment, Pinot Noir wines develop jammy and 'cooked' flavours that mask their elegance, complexity and silky qualities. The aromas vary from freshly crushed red fruit (particularly raspberries and strawberries), roses and spices (particularly sweet spices), to liquorice, well-hung game and farmyards, particularly as the wine ages.

The Pinot Noir wines are versatile with food. Their acidity makes them ideal with a wide range of fish, most meat (particularly game), pasta dishes and soft cheese that is not too pungent.

Cabernet Sauvignon

Cabernet Sauvignon seems to adapt itself to being successfully grown in most parts of the world. The associated aromas of wines which are predominantly Cabernet Sauvignon include blackcurrants, blackcurrant leaves, pencils, chocolate, cedar and cigar boxes. In the New World, the scents of eucalyptus, spices, herbs and green peppers can also be detected.

Cabernet Sauvignon may dominate in the Médoc in Bordeaux, although it will be blended with Merlot, Cabernet Franc and Petit Verdot. New World wines may use up to 95 per cent Cabernet Sauvignon in their blend and their makers do not have to declare the composition of the other 5 per cent. Generally, they will use a grape that benefits from blending, which produces a more complex and harmonious wine. Australia has produced good blends with the Syrah (Shiraz) grape, but generally Merlot is the favoured partner around the world.

These wines are good with red meat and hearty pasta dishes. Best served at room temperature.

Temperature and storage

Serve your white wines chilled, but not cold, to enable you to fully appreciate their flavours. Light-bodied reds like Beaujolais and dry rosés are also very refreshing in the summer when served chilled. Red wines should be served at room temperature and should be opened at least half an hour before they will be drunk so that oxygen has time to penetrate the wine and release a deeper flavour and aroma.

Wine should be stored in a dark room with a consistent temperature of between 10 and 16°C/50 and 60°F and a humidity level of 65–75 per cent. Because bottled wine can absorb the flavours around it, take care to store it in a place free from mould, mildew and household cleaners. Ideally, you should store your wine in a separate location of its own. The bottles should be positioned at an angle to keep the cork sufficiently moist and so prevent corkage problems.

food on the go

A picnic can be as simple as popping to your favourite delicatessen or as inspired as a black-tie champagne dinner, but find the right location and you will be transported to another world.

A day out by the sea, in the woods, on top of the roof, in your garden, at a friend's house or during your favourite sporting event can get your senses in tune with nature and restore your body and mind. Get away for a day. You will always remember it.

Keep it simple. Walk to your favourite vegetable market. Find the freshest fruit and vegetables – catch the scent of nature. Walk down the street until you can smell freshly baked bread. Go to your favourite cheese shop. Stop for a bottle of fresh, crisp wine. Or go all out. Plan a romantic day away and prepare all your favourite foods. Don't forget your camera.

Favourite picnics

I remember lazing in the sun with lots of friends eating some of my favourite foods. Think back to your most enjoyable picnic and plan another one today. Where did it take place and what did you eat? Remember what made it such fun – be inspired.

The South of France

Crusty French bread, Bleu d'Auvergne cheese, fresh tomatoes in season, red onion, Granny Smith apples and a crisp white wine.

Our patio

Freshly made hamburgers, blended ketchup/mustard sauce, potato salad, soft white rolls, brownies and fresh lemonade.

The Middle East

Pitta bread, houmous, fattosh salad, stuffed vine leaves, whole baby cucumbers, radishes, sweet yellow peppers, fresh figs and a bottle of Arak.

At the seaside

Soft-shell crab sandwiches, spicy collard greens, potato salad and ice-cold beer.

Up on the roof

Salade Niçoise, crusty French bread, fresh plums, goat's cheese and biscuits.

Going the distance

Make the day truly special by remembering all the small details. Presentation and careful food storage are as important as all the goodies that you've prepared.

Get out your favourite tablecloth and a nice blanket and pack your basket with all the essentials – china, glasses, cutlery, a bottle opener or corkscrew, a sharp knife, salt and pepper and serviettes. Don't forget about the sun and insects – throw in some sunscreen and repellents. Fill a Thermos with your favourite hot drink and another one with something cold.

An umbrella could always come in handy. Take your favourite book, a kite, a ball or Frisbee and play on the grass. Always clean up before you go so that someone else can enjoy the same spot.

The raw truth

Never put cooked foods on a platter with raw meat or chicken – and remember to clean your utensils after preparing raw meat before using them for anything else. If you are having a barbecue, always remember to cook chicken thoroughly, until the juices run clear and the meat is no longer pink.

When the sun beats down

On hot days, eat as soon as you get to your destination. The longer food sits out, the more likely bacteria are to flourish. You don't necessarily see, smell or taste when food has gone off. Be particularly careful with the food if there are infants or seniors on the picnic, or if there is anyone with a lowered immune system, as they could become dangerously ill. Invest in a good cooler. Pack both the bottom and the top of the cooler with ice. Keep it in a shady spot so it stays cold for as long as possible.

Chill out

For the most part, any fresh ingredient can spoil – from green salad to the icing on a cake, they can all suffer the effects of bacteria. Keep cool and be safe. Another good motto for life.

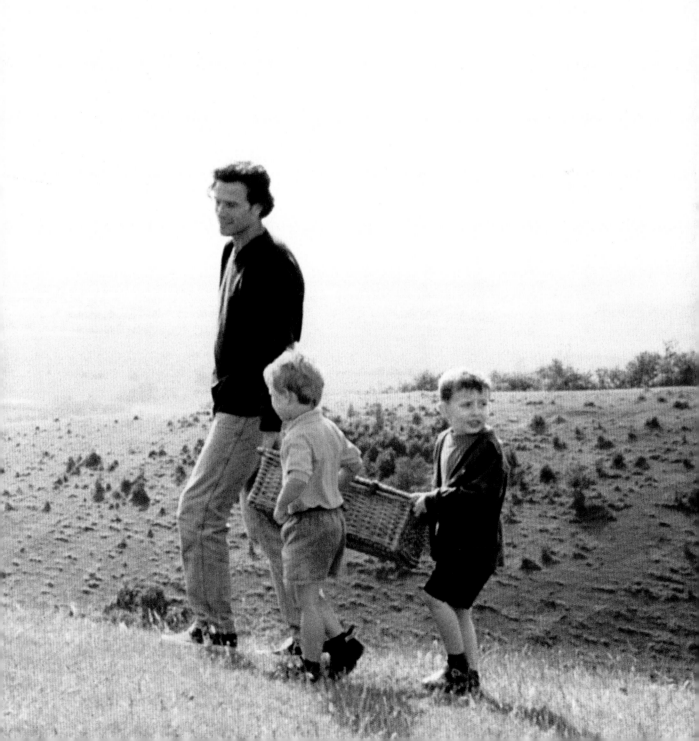

spending the night

If you have guests to stay for a night or more, try to be as welcoming as possible and give them all the comforts that they would have at home. Pay attention to the details in your guest's room and they will have a truly relaxing stay. How nice to be able to give your friends or family a well-deserved break!

I think that one must always have role models in life, and when I conjure up the perfect hostess, my friend Julie Dickinson comes to mind. My husband and I, along with a few odd poodles, go off and visit yearly to attend an annual theatre event. When we arrive, usually late afternoon, there is always a lovely tea, set outdoors when the weather permits. We always stay in the same room, which makes it very familiar, and it is always filled with everything we could possibly need.

There is a kettle with an assortment of herbal and traditional teas, coffee and a little jug of fresh milk and lovely biscuits to start the day at our own pace. There is fresh mineral water and glasses. An assortment of current magazines and newspapers as well as a radio are by the side of our bed. The bathroom is stacked with fresh towels and lovely scented soaps and all the toiletries we could require. We feel at home. We feel welcomed.

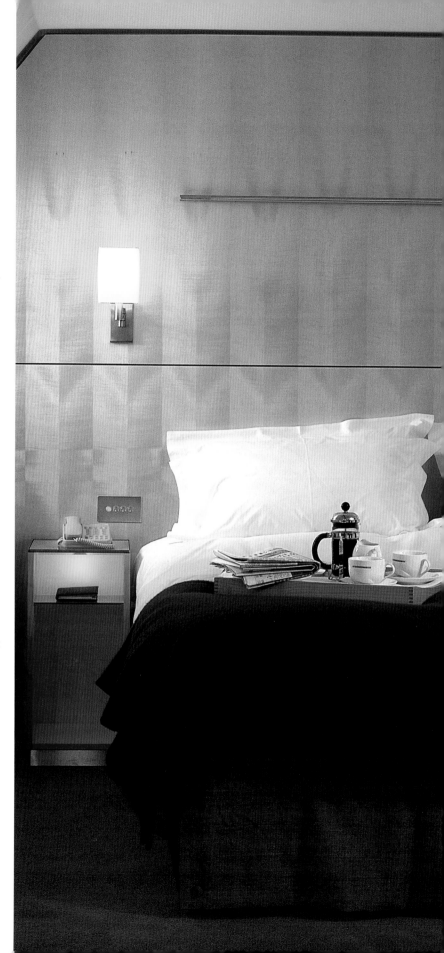

10 guest-room essentials

Acquaint your friends with the little-known facts and eccentricities of your house and encourage them to make themselves at home. Fill them in on what your usual morning is like and whether anything special has been planned for the day.

Give the room a good airing
Freshen up the room before your guests arrive. Throw open the windows to let the room breathe and allow air to circulate. Open the curtains and let the sun shine in.

Check the heating
In winter, make sure the radiators are turned on and the room is warm enough. Put a hot-water bottle in the bed several hours before your guests retire.

Create wardrobe space
Living out of a suitcase doesn't give you a sense of permanence. Leave the wardrobe door open and create some empty space for your guests with ample hangers.

Fill the room with flowers
Make the room inviting and seem lived in. Find some lovely scented flowers, like gardenias, lilies, freesia or lilacs, to give a feeling of friendliness and wellbeing.

Make up the bed with beautiful linen
Don't relegate your sorriest bedclothes to the guest room. Put on your favourite linen and duvet, with lots of plumped-up pillows.

Leave towels and soap
Stack your biggest bath towels, along with a face and hand towel, in the bedroom with fresh soap. Some bubble bath will give guests the hint that they are meant to relax.

Add some candles
Put some big, chunky scented candles by the bed, along with matches to light them. They can make the room feel special and are great in an emergency.

Stock up on refreshments
Leave some goodies for guests to nibble and drink. Fresh mineral water and glasses are a must. Tea and coffee with a kettle are pure luxury but are a lovely way to start the day.

Oops, I forgot
We all sometimes leave an essential item at home, so try to think about all the little things that your guests might need during their stay. Be discreet and place some potential comfort-savers in a basket. Shampoo, conditioner, toothpaste, cotton wool, aspirin and antacid, sanitary supplies and a spare loo roll will cover most situations. Your guests will know that you have taken the time to think of their comfort.

Inspire them
Leave some books or glossy magazines, or a radio or stereo with some favourite music, in the room for down-time. Make the room comfortable and relaxing.

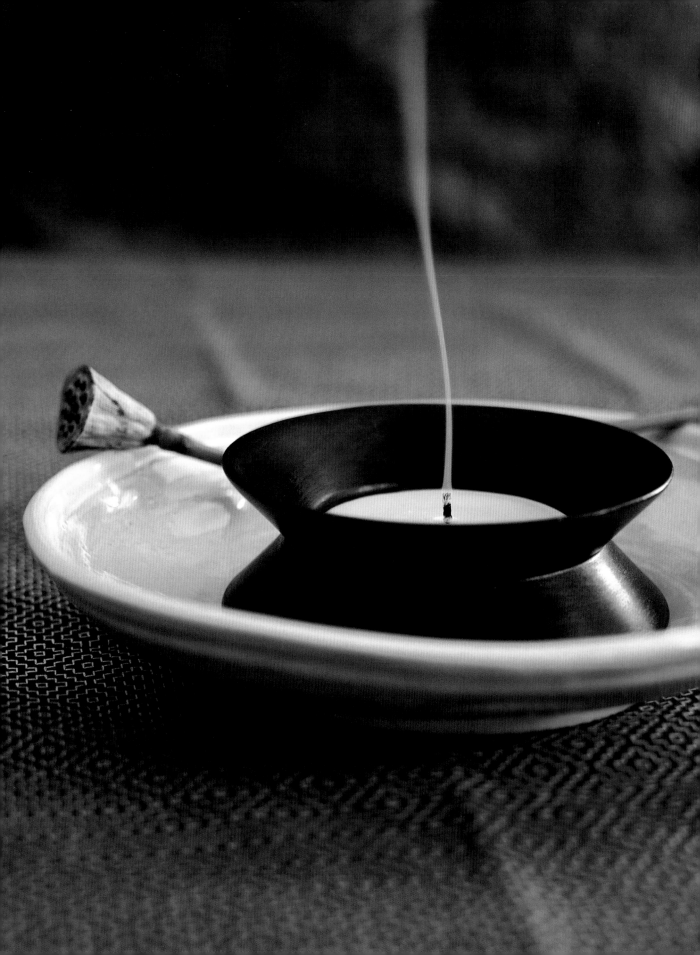

relaxation

"From time to time to remind ourselves to relax, to be peaceful, we may wish to set aside some time for a retreat, a day of mindfulness, when we walk slowly, smile, drink tea with a friend and enjoy being together as if we are the happiest people on the Earth." THICH NHAT HANH

Put on your favourite piece of music. Sit in your favourite chair and put your feet up. Close your eyes and listen. Take some deep breaths. Chill.

Relaxation is nourishment for your soul. It is the way that the body replenishes energy to get you through life's pressures. It is the light at the end of the tunnel. It's about balance.

Give yourself the time to relax and know how to enjoy it once you get it. This is the essence of getting a life. Plan relaxation as part of your daily routine, setting aside at least two hours a day to do something just for you. You'll find it will make you a more contented person. Your resentment at the pressures of work or family will slip away as you indulge yourself. You deserve your time. Don't ever forget that.

When you have your relaxation time is a matter of personal preference. Many people find that physical exercise is their greatest form of relaxation and will start the day by going to the gym or out into the fresh air for a run. Alternatively, a break at lunchtime can give you the extra energy to get through the day, particularly if you are able to take a walk outside. Others find that a big glass of wine while watching the television is the best way to kick back after a hard day at work. Whatever you choose to do and whenever you choose to do it are up to you. Just do it.

We all know people who seem to have a very difficult time relaxing, either because their mind is filled with worries because they feel unproductive if they are not being active. These people are in even more need of relaxation, as it is difficult to gain perspective if our mind and body never have a break.

Think about all the things that stimulate your senses. Beautiful sights, lovely fragrances and inspiring music can work wonders to help the body to wind down. Even something as simple as a room filled with lit candles creates a very peaceful atmosphere.

Give yourself treats, because you deserve them. Indulge yourself in your favourite ice cream, read a book from start to finish or soak in a hot tub just for the fun of it. Have a siesta in the middle of the day. Don't ever feel guilty about taking the time to do what you want.

Once you appreciate the calmness that you feel, you will know that this is the only way to live.

personal space

Meditation

Your surroundings are important in helping you to relax. Sitting in a bright, sunny room can change your attitude instantly. Many people get depressed during the winter months due to lack of sunlight. SAD (seasonal affective disorder) is a light-deprivation disorder that affects mainly women and causes recurrent, cyclical bouts of depression and tiredness. In Scandinavia, which has very limited sunlight during winter months, many cities have developed 'light rooms' which use artificial lights to re-create the sun's spectrum. People just pop in to get some light therapy. It works! So let the light into your home or get outside and make the most of the sunshine.

My relaxation is as simple as a walk in the park each morning with my dogs. Rain or shine, it is one of the most pleasurable experiences of my day. I watch the mist rising from the ponds and see the swans and ducks swimming with their young. I smell the honeysuckle from a distance and am intoxicated by the beauty of nature in the middle of a bustling city. My dogs run free and meet up with their friends to socialise, which makes them very happy and friendly pets. I am inspired and relaxed. I gain a sense of perspective as nature goes about its business. It is pure bliss. I am home by 8.30am to start my day with a new lease of life.

Think about how you feel after a restless night's sleep. I know that if I haven't slept properly I feel exhausted and unable to focus clearly the following day. Lack of relaxation can make you go through your days with a low battery.

Over the years, when I have had restless times, I have tried various forms of meditation to help restore the balance in my hectic life. It doesn't have to be complicated – just a little time on your own to be quiet and still. As little as fifteen minutes a day meditating can really make a difference.

We also need some personal time and space to collect our thoughts. If you share a space with your family, designate a time of the day and a room that is strictly your own.

Quieten your mind

Relax your body

15 minutes a day

Sit in your favourite chair or out in the open air

Close your eyes

Concentrate on your breathing

Exhale to the count of four

Inhale to the count of four

Slow down

Listen to your breathing

Concentrate on one word

If your mind wanders, bring it back

One word

Relax

Be quiet

15 minutes in the grand scale of life

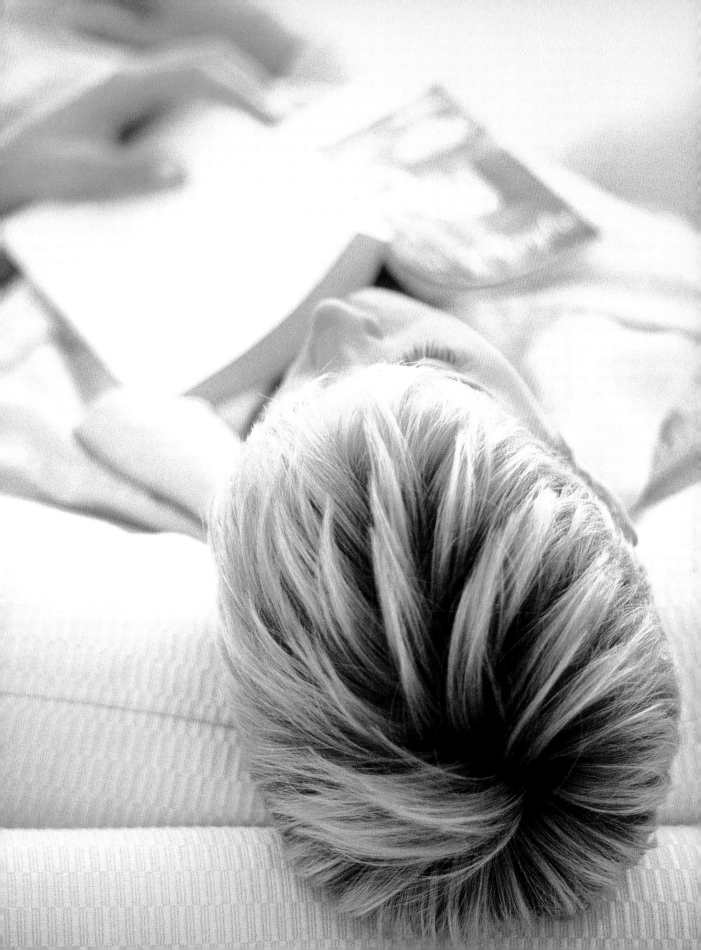

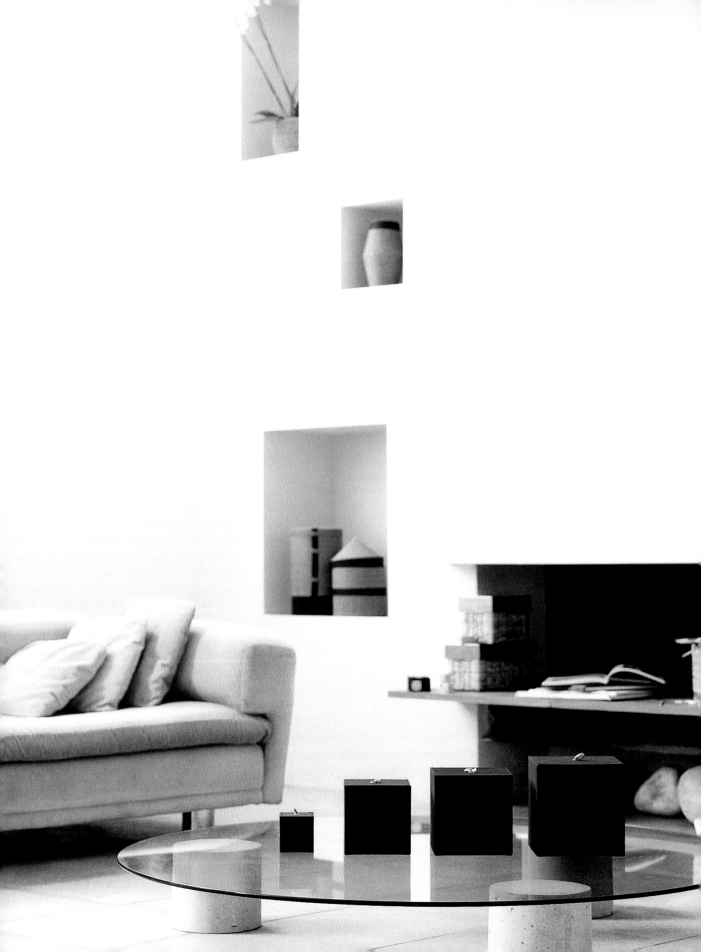

making time for relaxation

In a perfect world we wouldn't have to worry about making the time to relax. We would be relaxed all of the time. Think about what you could achieve if the fears, anxieties and frenetic feelings that you have some of the time were gone. What if every day felt like you were on holiday? Wouldn't it be fabulous? It would make everything more simple and much easier to cope with. We would be happier in what we do and we would achieve more.

Let's pretend

Close your eyes and imagine that you are on your favourite holiday. Re-create in your mind what you were wearing and what the weather was like. Think about how you spent your time. Did you catch up on lost sleep or get up early and watch the sunrise? Did you lie around on a beach soaking up the sun or explore the areas around you? How did you feel? Did you notice the colours and the smells? Did you enjoy your meals? Can you picture them now? Did you leave your worries behind, knowing that they weren't that important? Did you lose the sense of time altogether by just taking things as they came along? Did you forget what day of the week it was? Did you talk more? Did you laugh more? If you can do it on holiday, you can do it every day – no matter where you are.

When we are on holiday, we tend to appreciate the act of getting away, or having a break. We mentally lock the door of our mind to the things that worry us and make a fresh start. We set out to have a good time because we know that we deserve it. And very importantly, we make the most of every minute of our time away.

Practice makes perfect

Every day, whether you are at work or doing things around the house, give yourself a relaxing break, even if it is just for five minutes. Do it throughout the day. Simply pretend that you are on holiday. Close your eyes, kick back and recreate the feeling. The more you are able to put yourself in a relaxed state, the more you will enjoy everything that you do. It really can and will make a difference to your life.

Relaxation stimulates all of your senses. You become more aware of the things around you. You perceive how things feel, look and smell. You do things because you enjoy them. Your body knows how to relax if only you give it the right signals to do so.

Think about the difference between eating food on the run and going over to a friend's house for dinner. You probably can't remember what you had for lunch the other day but could re-create all aspects of the dinner party. The difference is that you were not taking the time to relax and appreciate one and were completely at ease and relaxed for the other.

Home and away

We all know the benefits of getting away. Do it more often. It doesn't have to be a fortnight away at your favourite beach resort. A weekend or even a night away can make all the difference. We can all do with a change of scenery. Just having something to look forward to will change your outlook on life. You have the power to do it. Take control and see how much better you feel. Make space for free time.

Every now and again plan a weekend away right in your very own home. If you have children, arrange for them to stay with family or friends. Turn on the answer machine and pretend that you are off to your favourite destination. Indulge yourself in all the luxuries you secretly dream about. Sleep in, read lots of books, turn your bathroom into a health spa and try all of your favourite beauty treatments. Turn off the outside world and you will come back feeling like a whole new person.

10 ways to indulge at home

Simulate your senses. Smell the roses. Be creative. Paint your toenails. Think about what really makes you feel wonderful and just do it. These are my favourite things.

Fill your house with flowers

Lift your spirits with a burst of colour. Put them next to your bed, by your favourite chair and by the bath. Make your eyes smile.

Have a long soak in the tub

Get out your favourite bath products and run a very hot bath. Stay in until your fingers start to wrinkle. Soak away your worries.

Light some candles

Surround yourself with light. Choose scented candles and soak it all in. Meditate, pray or just sit in peace. Indulge your spirituality.

Catch up on your sleep

Turn off your alarm clock and get those batteries fully charged. Wake up when your body tells you it's ready and not a minute before. Stay in bed for as long as you like.

Rent your favourite videos

Have a movie marathon in your own home. Get the videos that really make you laugh or cry. Veg out in front of the telly, put your feet up and let those emotions go.

Eat your favourite food

Indulge your taste buds by getting all of your favourite foods. Be it a tub of ice cream or a jar of caviar, relish every last morsel. Don't think about the calories.

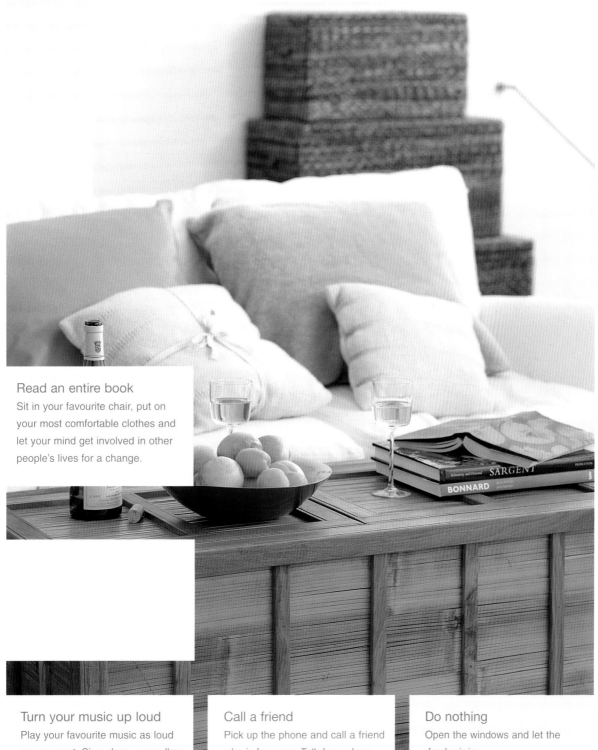

Read an entire book
Sit in your favourite chair, put on your most comfortable clothes and let your mind get involved in other people's lives for a change.

Turn your music up loud
Play your favourite music as loud as you want. Sing along, regardless of whether you can carry a tune. It is really liberating.

Call a friend
Pick up the phone and call a friend who is far away. Talk for as long as you want. Don't think about how much it costs. Let time fly.

Do nothing
Open the windows and let the fresh air in.
Breathe…
Do absolutely nothing.

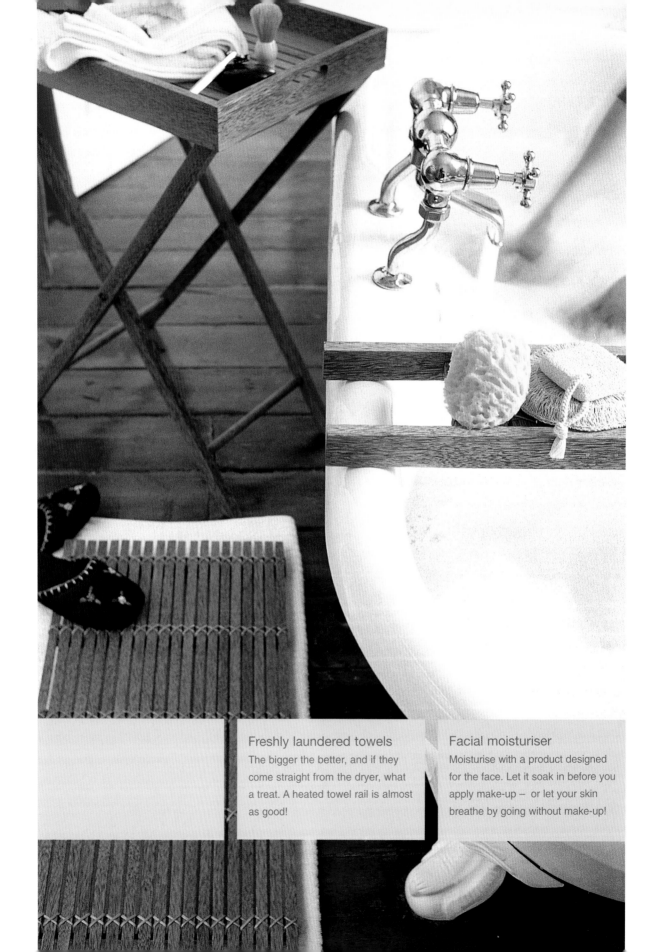

Freshly laundered towels

The bigger the better, and if they come straight from the dryer, what a treat. A heated towel rail is almost as good!

Facial moisturiser

Moisturise with a product designed for the face. Let it soak in before you apply make-up — or let your skin breathe by going without make-up!

10 ways to have a luxurious bath

For the most relaxing night in the world, really treat yourself to an indulgent bath. Get all your favourite scented products. Take your time. Splash around.

Treat your feet
We pound them and squeeze them into tiny shoes. A pumice foot scrub used weekly will keep them soft and feeling their best.

Exfoliating brush
Get rid of all your skin's debris and get your circulation moving with a good exfoliating brush. Don't forget to scrub your back!

Scented bubble bath
Have a giggle with a bath full of fragrant bubbles. Close your eyes and inhale.

Skin-polishing mitt
You polish the silver, now polish your skin! Give yourself a natural glow with a soft skin-polishing mitt.

Scented body lotion
Keep a selection on hand to trap the moisture and keep you smelling fresh. Match your favourite scent with the same-fragrance body lotion.

Dead Sea salts
Dead Sea salts relax stiff muscles and calm and soothe your soul.

Talcum powder
When you were a baby, your mother always took the time to powder you after bathing. Try using a big, fluffy puff and your favourite powder.

Scented candle
Always set an indulgent mood before you bathe.

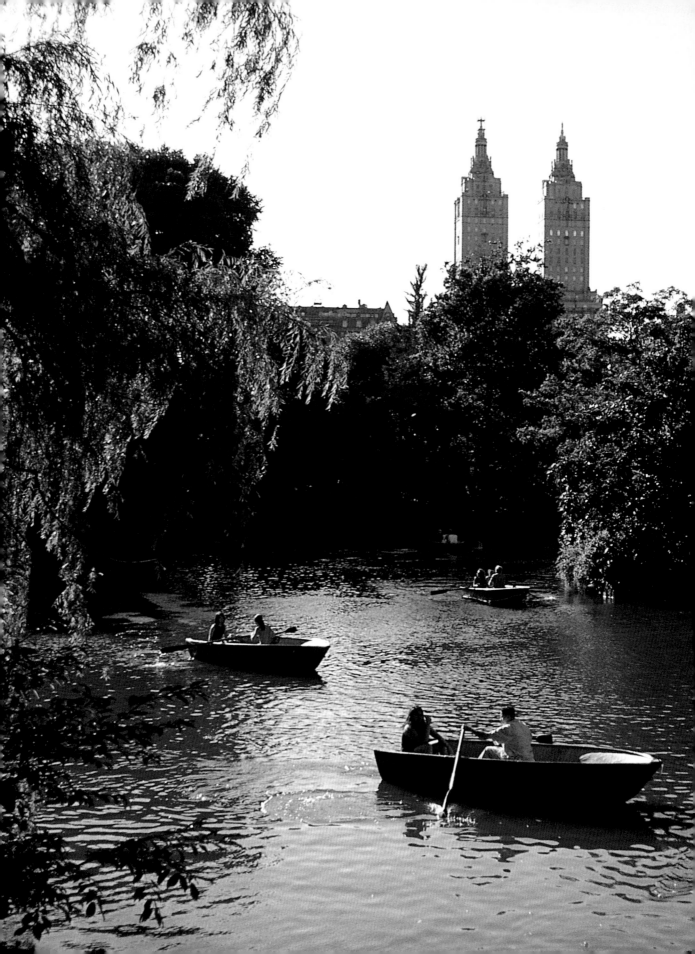

the great outdoors

No matter what your schedule is like, take some time each day to go outdoors and enjoy the natural elements.

It sounds so simple. We all go outside every day for various reasons, but most of the time we are in our own little world, oblivious of everything around us. We think too much. Why not make it a point to really pay attention to what is going on around you? Watch the people and make eye contact. Smile. Be connected. Get ideas. Look at what people are reading. See how they dress or wear their hair. Soak it all in.

Look in shop windows. Catch the scent of perfume, flowers or food that may be lingering in the air. Remember them. Take in the colours. Form opinions. Sit outside and have a coffee or relax on a bench and read the paper. Feel the sun. Listen to the rain. Be a sponge. Absorb everything.

Get grounded

When you are having a hard time finding your footing, plant your feet firmly on the ground and get digging. Don't wear gloves – feel the earth between your fingers. It's a great way to channel excess energy. If you are lucky enough to have a garden, tend it every day. You will be amazed how good it feels. You will start to gain a keen awareness of how things change all the time. If you don't have the space, plant a window box, grow herbs in your kitchen or scatter potted plants around.

Take a walk on the wild side

The next time you are thinking of going somewhere in your car, walk instead. Gain a different point of view. See how many places you can shop in your own neighbourhood. Support your local businesses. Walk fast for 20 minutes and get your exercise. You'll meet your neighbours and you'll save the environment by using less fuel.

Make a picnic

On the next nice weekend day, have a picnic. Be spontaneous. Grab some bread and cheese and a bottle of wine and find a running stream or beautiful meadow. Take a nice wool blanket and lie on the grass, soaking up the rays. Stretch your body and your mind. Lie on your back and look up at the sky.

Go for a jog

Get those endorphins moving and clear your mind. Take a half-hour jog several days a week. Push yourself. Get the blood flowing. Take different routes. Look at everything that is going on around you. Breathe deeply. Perspire. Get rid of toxins.

Row, row, row your boat gently down the stream

Get the Sunday papers and find your closest body of water with boats to rent. Row out to a peaceful spot, moor the boat and read the papers. Let the water gently move you. What could be better?

Collect seashells

Take a walk on the beach at any time of the year. Bring along your dogs or kids and play Sand Olympics. Make up the rules as you go along. Take your shoes off, roll up your trousers and stick your feet in the water. Don't worry about the cold. Do a cartwheel. Make a castle. Keep a memento and think about your day away whenever you look at it.

Swim with the fish

Find the nearest outdoor pool and go for a swim. Listen to your breathing. Count your lengths. Change your strokes. Play water volleyball. Take the plunge.

Go out to play

Do what you did when you were a kid. Call up your friends and see if they can come out to play. Have a game of football. Play tennis or crazy golf. Go roller-blading. Do it as a group. Be competitive. Try your hardest. Have fun.

Ride a bicycle

My dear friend Celia says that riding a bike is just like life. You have many uphill struggles and then there is the easy bit, when it takes no effort at all. Try a circular route where the uphill and downhill balance out. Just like life.

Do nothing

Have a siesta in your favourite green space. Listen to the birds. Smell the flowers. Be at peace.

working out

If physical exercise is undertaken regularly – three to five times a week for at least 45 minutes – it will change your life. It will boost your stamina, give you more energy, make you feel and look better, make you more confident and, in general, make you a much better person to be around. You will realise that you have a life and a body that are worth looking after.

It can be difficult to find the time to take regular exercise, particularly in these times of long working days, but when you do find the time to establish a regular workout routine, the benefits are countless. If you can't exercise in the mornings before heading to the office and you feel that you may miss out on seeing your friends in the evenings, get them to enrol in a class with you. Make it a regular event. Do a dance class, like salsa or jazz, to make it really fun. You'll meet new people and have a great time while giving your mind and your body a well-earned energy boost.

Smarten up

Exercise increases blood flow to the brain, stimulating your mental activity and your ability to learn. It also has been shown to increase your memory. Couldn't we all use a boost in the brain department? Why not start every day with 30 minutes of physical exercise and give yourself a brain vitamin? While you're at it, practise posing a question to your mind and asking for the solution at the beginning of your fitness routine. Forget about it when you are working out. Write down what comes into your head when you have finished. Utilise that freshly stimulated brain. You won't know whether it works unless you try it.

Heart and soul

Aerobic exercise is considered the most effective for keeping your heart, lungs and circulatory system in tip-top condition. Aerobic exercise moves oxygen throughout your body, and oxygen in turn nourishes your tissues and balances your body chemistry.

To train aerobically, you need to get your heart, lungs and circulatory system working together at an elevated rate for about 20 minutes. You can calculate your pulse rate, or get to know your body by looking for the following signs: faster but not laboured breathing, an awareness of your heart beating but not pounding and you may begin to perspire. When you get to where you are working at optimum levels, feel the flow from the release of the chemical beta-endorphin from your brain that causes a feeling of general wellbeing. This is good for the soul. Aerobic exercise does not have to take place in a gym. Power-walking, running, cycling or anything that gets that heart pumping will do the trick.

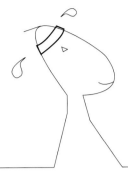

Build up your strength

Strength training conditions and strengthens the muscles, bones and connective tissues and is especially important for women of a certain age to help ward off osteoporosis, the weakening of the bones that can happen after menopause. You don't have to build big muscles to achieve the benefits of this type of exercise.

Strength training is accomplished by any activity in which your muscles contract against an applied resistance. In a gym, this is done with free weights, weight-training machines or with exercises such as callisthenics or certain types of yoga. It's best done in a gym with proper supervision. Make sure to tell the instructor what you wish to achieve with your strength training – basic conditioning or bulkier muscles. They will help design a programme to achieve your goals.

Be flexible

'Stay loose, Mother Goose' is a great saying of my friend Kate. It pretty much sums up life. Be flexible in your attitude and in your body to eliminate emotional and physical stresses from your life.

Practise flexibility every day. Stretch your body and your mind. You don't have to win every battle. You don't have to enter the marathon. Go with the flow. Increase the range of muscle motion in your joints to prevent you from injuring yourself during exercise. Stretch daily.

Yoga is a perfect way to stretch both your mind and your body. Its movements flow with the breath to balance the physical and mental and release a sense of calm. There are different forms of yoga, all of which follow the same basic principles, so seek out the right one for you. Try a few different classes to find one where you feel that you can learn, stretch yourself and, above all, relax. Don't rush. Take your time. Keep an open mind.

Get addicted

It is said that to truly make something a habit, it takes six weeks of constant repetition. If you're not enjoying the exercise routine you've planned then it will be difficult to stick to. If you really don't enjoy sweating it out in a gym or if you're not cut out for yoga, then get outside – start jogging, ask your friends to join you in a regular football game or set the pace and start walking. Establish a routine that you enjoy and make it a part of your day. Get through the six weeks and you will miss not doing it, even for a day. Get high on life.

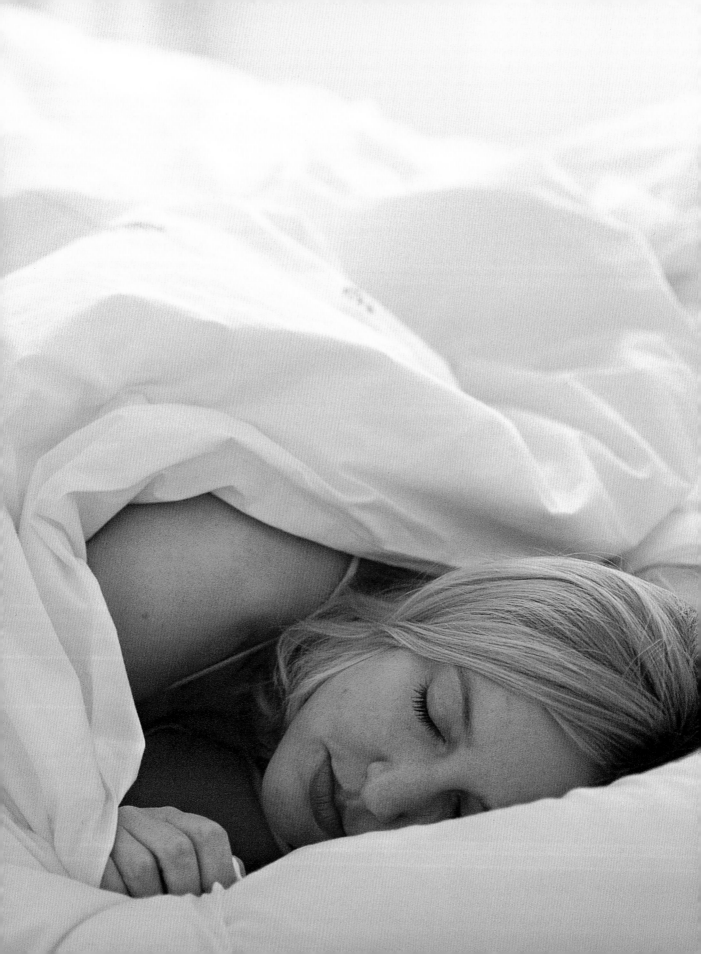

bedtime

Getting a good night's sleep makes you feel and look better. Dark circles under the eyes are not an attractive sight. How much sleep you need depends on you. Your body will tell you if you get too much or too little. Too little will make it difficult to get through the next day and too much can make you sluggish in the morning. Some 60 per cent of the population sleep between six and eight hours a night. Think about how much sleep you require to feel at your best.

Many things can impact on whether we have a good night's rest. Tension or stress is one of the leading causes of lack of sleep. The more you worry about it, the less likely you are to fall asleep. Don't force yourself. If you can't sleep, get out of bed and read a book.

If you are prone to restless nights there are things that you can do during the day to avoid problems. Take half an hour of exercise each day. A walk after dinner can help you to digest your meal so that your body is ready to sleep at bedtime. Avoid too much caffeine during the day: it may give you a buzz, but it can also set you on edge. Keep alcohol consumption within moderation as it can cause interrupted sleep.

As with everything, develop a bedtime routine and it will become a natural part of the day. Try to go to bed at about the same time every night. Your body will naturally get sleepy as you approach bedtime. Give your face a good scrub or get into a relaxing bath. Pamper yourself. Set aside a few

minutes to think about your day. Ask yourself whether you achieved what you had hoped, and if not, how you would change tomorrow to learn from today.

Keep a journal. It doesn't have to be long. Write down three things that you were thankful for during the day and anything special or inspiring. Somehow writing it down gives it importance.

Make sure that your bedroom is not stuffy. Open the windows and let some fresh air in. Do some deep breathing while sitting comfortably with your eyes closed. Let your thoughts go and relax.

Look around you. Make sure you have what you need at your fingertips. Think about whatever will relax you, make you smile and get you into the right mood for the sweetest of dreams.

be a sleeping beauty

Why we require sleep still remains a medical mystery, but we all know how we feel when we don't get enough of it. Maintaining your energy levels throughout the day and looking good can be achieved only after a proper night's rest. Your friends will be the first to tell you that you look tired, even when you may not feel it.

According to research by the US National Commission on Sleep Disorders, one in every three people on any given night has difficulty falling or staying asleep. If you take it a step further, one in every three people is not at their best the next day. Pay attention to the signs. Keep track of the periods of the day when you can't stop yawning or have very low energy levels to help you determine whether you are getting the proper rest.

There is only so much overdraft or sleep debt that the body's bank will allow. Because of the stimulating effects the light and our environment have on us, we may not know it. A sleep debt can become so great that we cannot resist falling asleep, sometimes in potentially dangerous situations like when driving a car.

We all have different sleep patterns and need different amounts of sleep, so it could be that too much sleep for you is not enough for others. Your body will give you the signs – listen to it.

Sleep patterns

If you have a difficult time getting to sleep, keeping a sleep diary over a period of 1–2 weeks can help you to analyse what is causing it and whether you are accumulating a sleep debt.

Before you go to bed, write down the time and how sleepy you feel using a scale of 1–10, 10 being the sleepiest. Write down any particular worries you may have and what foods you ate during the day. When you awake, write down when you think you fell asleep, whether you got up during the night and what time you awoke. Think about whether you were woken by light or noise and whether you were hot or cold. All these factors influence your sleep patterns.

If you find that your energy levels are high and your concentration is normal despite sleeping problems, then you are a rare individual who can survive with less rest. It may not last for ever. Most of us require seven and a half hours of sleep to feel well rested. Only 2 per cent of the population can get by with five hours. The older we get, the more sleep our bodies require.

If you find that you are sleepy during the day and have less energy than you need, your body needs more rest. Read your diary and look for common themes that may be contributing to your restless nights.

If you have a difficult time getting to sleep, keeping a sleep diary over a period of 1–2 weeks can help you to analyse what is causing it. . .

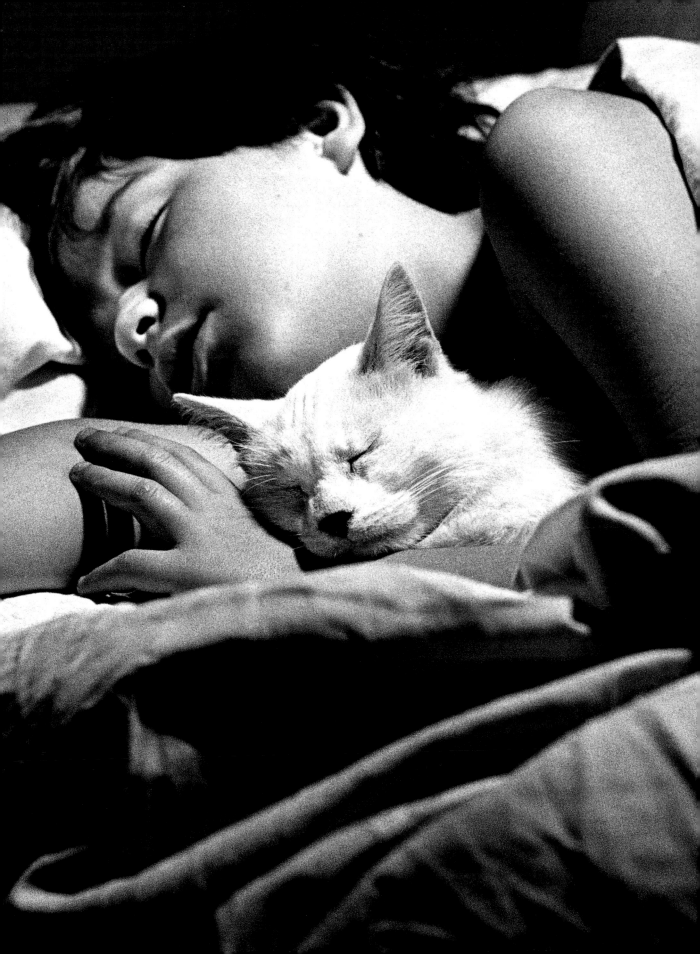

10 ways to get a great night's sleep

1

You are what you eat
Heavy foods in the evening can make you wake feeling bloated. Try eating your evening meal a little earlier and stay away from rich or greasy foods late in the day.

2

Bathing beauty
Soak away the stresses of the day with a hot bath using essential oils. Let your mind wander where it wants to go. Moisturise all over and wrap yourself in a bathrobe. Sit quietly in your favourite chair for 10 minutes and relax.

3

Water baby
Before going to sleep, drink a large glass of water. It helps to flush the impurities from your system, particularly if you have over-indulged with food or drink.

4

Ray of sunshine
Try leaving the curtains or blinds in your bedroom open before going to sleep to allow the morning light to awaken you. This is a great way to get your body attuned to the natural rhythms of the season.

5

Mask it out
For a refreshing treat, sleep with a cool gel mask over your eyes to reduce puffiness. If you don't have an eye mask, keep a bottle of your favourite toner or astringent in the refrigerator and dampen cotton wool pads with the cool toner. Close your eyes and place the pads over them for 10 minutes before going to bed. Listen to your breathing and relax.

6 Breeze through

Sleep with the windows open a little, regardless of the time of year. It will stop the room feeling stuffy and will counter the effects of any heating or air conditioning.

7 Chill out

Sleep with the minimal amount of covers and clothing to feel comfortable. Too many bedclothes can cause the body to overheat during the night and you may wake up with a headache.

8 Silent night

If the slightest sound wakes you up then try sleeping with foam ear-plugs to block out any unwanted disturbances.

9 Music maestro

If you have a radio or stereo with a timer in your bedroom, try lulling yourself to sleep at night, and waking yourself up in the morning, to some soothing classical music. Begin and end your day a calmer way.

10 Positive thinking

Remember all the great things that happened today. Think of all the things that you look forward to doing tomorrow.

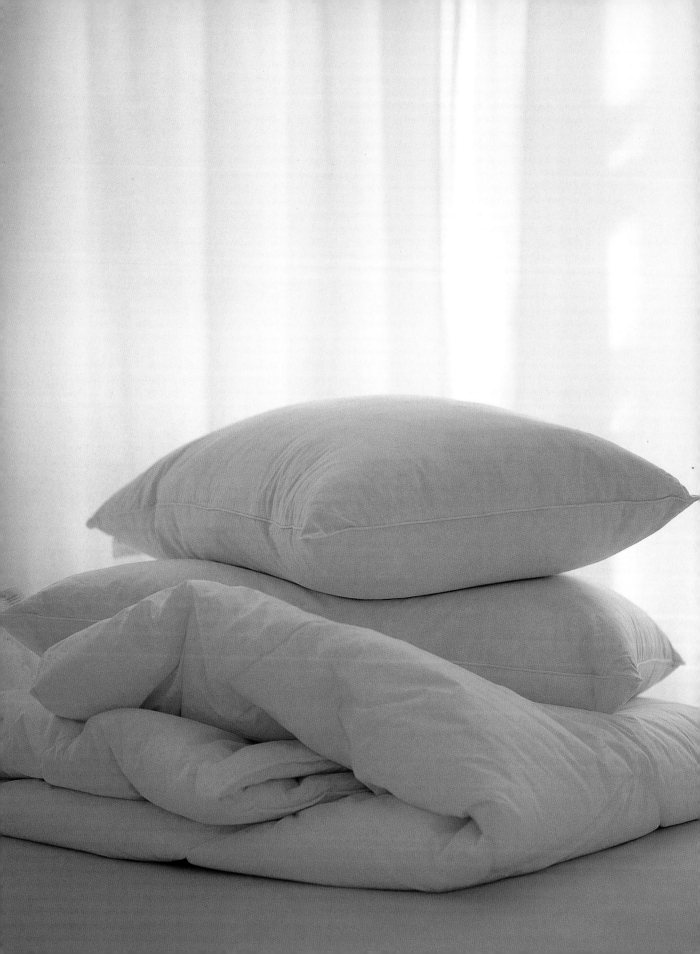

lying in comfort

Most people change where they live and what they drive more often than their mattress or pillows. Nothing lasts for ever. A good mattress should last about 10 years.When is the last time you replaced your mattress? Don't wait until you find yourself rolling into the middle of the bed when you turn over or being pinched in the back by a broken spring to buy a new one. The chances are that you're not getting the benefits of a good night's sleep and you wake up feeling stiff. As soon as you hear the mattress start to creak, change it.

Building a foundation

The most important way to judge a mattress is by how it feels. When buying a mattress, ignore the manufacturer's description and the salesperson's pitch – take off your shoes and lie on it. If the mattress is too soft it will give way to your lower back, if it's too firm there will be too much pressure on your hips, back and shoulders. If your partner likes a different firmness of mattress to you, buy one with two different sides.

Take your time. A third of your life is spent sleeping. Although there are very few studies showing the effects of a good mattress on how well you sleep, ask anyone who complains of back pain how their mattress affects them and you will invest in the best. Being comfortable and relaxed are prerequisites for a good sleep.

Pillow talk

Choosing the right pillow is essential if you want to get a good night's sleep. They come in a variety of sizes, shapes and materials to suit all sleep habits and accommodate all bed sizes. Remember, though, that American and European sizes vary.

The best pillows, which are unfortunately also the most expensive, are made from prime goose down and make you feel like you are drifting off to sleep on a cloud. The benefits of down pillows are that they are extremely lightweight and long-lasting. A friend of mine has her pillows made in a tiny town in Alsace, France. She actually goes to select the feathers and swears that they are the finest pillows in the world. Wherever she travels, she always takes her pillow with her.

Feather pillows are a cheaper version of down, being the least expensive type that you can buy. They are more firm than down and come in a variety of weights. Test them out to make sure that there are no sharp edges poking through.

You can also get pillows with a combination of feathers for firmness and down for softness which come at a middle-of-the-road price.

For those with allergies, it may be best to use polyester pillows, which are available in different degrees of firmness. The best quality polyester pillows can be expensive.

Foam pillows are another option for those with allergies. Make sure that the foam is of the best quality or it will deteriorate more quickly than pillows made with other materials.

As a general rule of thumb (although only your body knows for sure), firm pillows are usually best for people who sleep on their side, soft pillows work better for those who sleep on their tummy and medium pillows give the right support for those who sleep on their back.

Always put a cover on your pillow before putting on your pillowcase. It can help extend the life of your pillow and keep it free from the natural oils on your scalp. Wash the pillow cover along with your bedlinen weekly.

When buying a mattress, ignore the... salesperson's pitch – take off your shoes and lie on it.

the well-dressed bed

The well-dressed bed should always be ready for any occasion. Be prepared for the onset of sweet dreams or for more intimate moments by taking the time first thing each morning to make your bed look perfect. Fold your blankets. Plump your pillows. Straighten your sheets and duvet. Get rid of the clutter. Spray some lavender water under the covers to keep them fresh.

Cotton on

Invest in the best sheets you can afford. You don't have to have lots of sets, three will do. I would gladly sacrifice one set to have truly beautiful, luxurious cotton sheets. Choose the very best cotton, even if you have to iron them, as they really improve with age. Check the weave. The denser the thread-count, the better.

In the quest for an easy-care world, many bedclothes are manufactured in synthetic blends of polyester and cotton. Although it reduces the need for ironing, these just don't hold a candle to the beauty of natural fibres that breathe and keep you cool. Be adventurous. Try linen in the summer, cotton flannel in the winter or satin when it strikes your fancy. Indulge in a selection of different colours to adjust to the seasonal lighting or just to pick up your mood.

Cover up

The covers you choose to keep you warm will depend on the season.

Duvets or quilts come in a variety of weights and fillings to make you comfortable all year. Feather is the warmest while still being lightweight, but there are many synthetic fillings that can be used in all temperatures as well.

Blankets or shawls are an added sign of cosiness and are great to throw around your shoulders when snuggled up with your favourite book. Try merino wool, which is the softest to the touch, or polar fleece, a modern, synthetic fabric that is very warm and available in a great selection of patterns and colours. In the summer, use just a top sheet or a lightweight cotton cover.

Making up

How you make your bed is a matter of personal choice. I use both a fitted sheet and top sheet and then have a duvet on top. I would rather launder a top sheet than a duvet cover on a weekly basis. Some prefer to forgo the extra top sheet in favour of having just a duvet, which will then require washing more often.

Ideally, it is lovely to hang your linen outside to dry and iron sheets and covers when still a bit damp. If you give them a good tug before you hang them, you may get away without ironing at all. If you must use a dryer, do so on a low setting and remove while still a bit damp to the touch to iron more easily. Always find the time to keep your duvet looking wrinkle-free.

Bedlinen sizing varies greatly around the world. Before you go out to buy new sheets, take the dimensions of the mattress and don't forget to measure the thickness, as many fitted sheets will not fit extra-thick mattresses. Standard mattress thicknesses are between 17 and 20cm/7 and 8 in.

All dressed up

Beautiful sheets and bedcovers have been passed down through families for generations. Often they were part of the wedding trousseau, so special care was taken to select the finest cottons and linens that would withstand the test of time. Many cultures delicately embroider the finest cotton sheets as a special gift and families gather in many parts of the world to assemble a quilted bedcover as a symbol of good luck for the married couple. Many antique shops stock supplies of lovely old bedlinen. Shop around and you could find the perfect complement to your bed.

Your well-dressed bed should invite and entice you. It should beckon you for a snooze on a sunny afternoon and soothe you after a day of hard work. It should feel comfortable – the firmness of the mattress and fluffiness of the pillows; the smoothness of the sheets and warmth of the duvet. Take the time every morning to give it some special attention. Like an old friend, it will be waiting to nurture, comfort and protect you. Sweet dreams.

Use this quick reference chart to help select the proper linen size for your bed: all dimensions are given in inches.

The mattress type on the left is the European name, followed by its American description.

European		Mattress type	American	
Fitted	Flat		Fitted	Flat
36 x 75	70 x 102	Single / Twin	39 x 75	70 x 96
54 x 75	90 x 102	Double / Full	54 x 75	72 x 108
60 x 78	106 x 108	King / Queen	60 x 80	90 x 102
72 x 78	118 x 105	Super King / King	72 x 80	108 x 120

keeping a journal

10 things to keep next to the bed

A great reading lamp.

A notebook and pen.

Fresh mineral water and a pretty glass.

A photograph.

A plant or fresh flowers.

A scented candle.

Essential oils to help you sleep.

A handkerchief or tissues.

A favourite book.

An alarm clock.

Oprah Winfrey said in a television interview that each day she wrote down six things to be grateful for. What an inspirational thing to do every day. By taking the time to look for the positive things that occur each day we can only attract more positive things to us. It changes your outlook on life. Accentuate the positive and eliminate the negative. Saying thank you is one of the greatest lessons we can learn. Do you always remember to be thankful, even for the little things? Try it more often. It changes people's attitude towards you in an instant. Think about it.

Keeping a journal is a great way to wind down the day. Do it at the same time every day and it will become part of you. Bedtime is the right time for me. It puts closure on the day and gives me insight. Take the time to learn the lessons that life brings each day and you will grow. If we don't learn from our mistakes, we are destined to repeat them.

Start with the six things you give thanks for and remind yourself why you are happy to be you. List the things that inspired you during the day. Think about them and be inspired all over again. If you did not take the time to be inspired, what got in the way? Write it down. If you are inspired, it will rub off on everything you do. Everyone you come into contact with will feel the energy and be inspired to do greater things. Don't dwell on the bad stuff.

Be brief. Write it down. Think about it. Always make the first move to change something negative, regardless of the situation behind it.

From time to time take a look back at the journals you have kept. Do the same things continue to make you happy? If so, try to re-create these feelings more throughout each day. If you find that you are still frustrated by the same things, confront them. Look at the past, but don't dwell on it. Think about the future, but don't live in it. Take each day as it comes. Write it down. It is who you are.

Saying thank you is one of the greatest lessons we can learn. Do you always remember to be thankful, even for the little things?

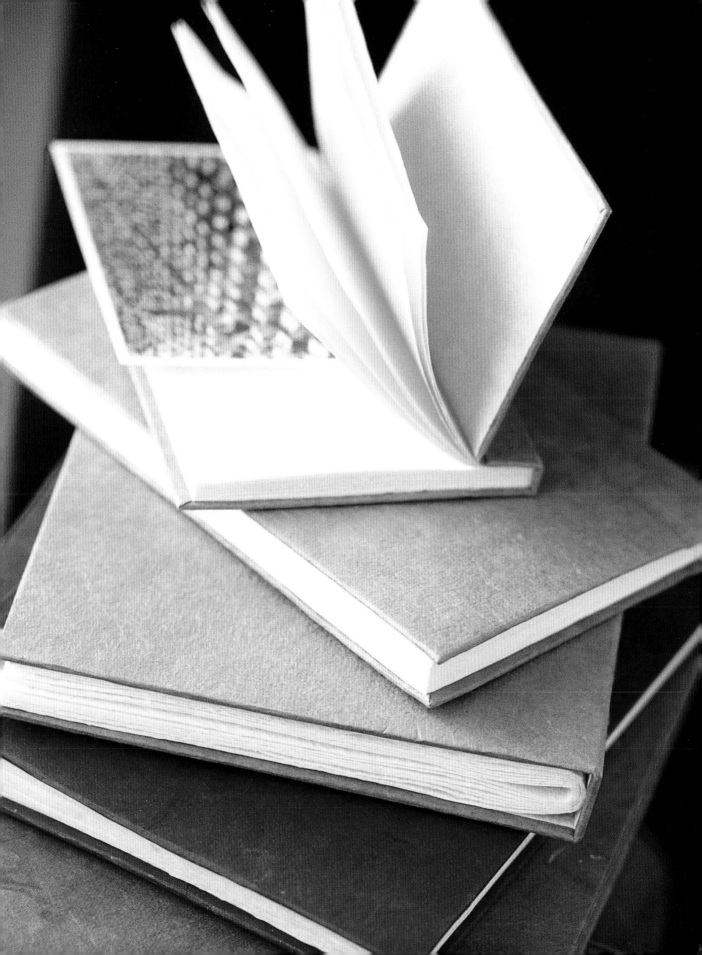

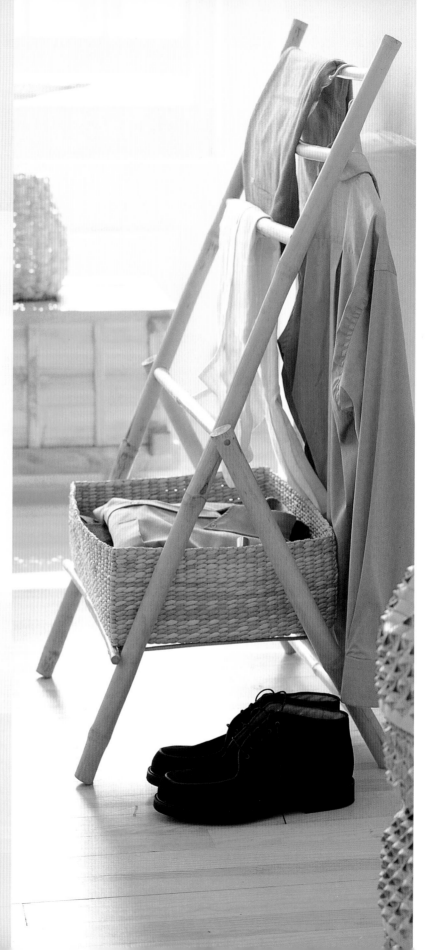

10 things
to do
before you
go to bed

Hang up all the clothes
you wore today.

Lay out your clothes
for tomorrow.

Make a list of what you
hope to achieve tomorrow.

Write in your journal.

Allow 10 minutes for a
thorough cleansing of your face
– don't forget to moisturise.

Always floss your teeth –
they will come in handy in
your later years.

Throw away all the papers that
have accumulated in your room.

Read an inspirational book for
15 minutes.

Set your alarm clock.

Say your prayers, meditate or
lie quietly to reflect on the day.

books at bedtime

There are some books that, no matter how many times you read them, continue to provide comfort and uplift your soul. When the stresses and strains of daily life get to you, read some of these bedtime stories to inspire your dreams.

The Alchemist
Paulo Coelho

Meditations for
Women Who Do Too Much
Ann Wilson Schaef

Tuesdays with Morrie
Mitch Albom

Titania's Wishing Spells:
Health, Wealth,
Love, Happiness
Titania Hardie

Talking to Heaven:
A Medium's Message
of Life After Death
James Van Praagh

Don't Sweat the Small
Stuff and It's All Small Stuff
Richard Carlson

The Pilgrimage
Paulo Coelho

Conversations
with God – Book One
Neale Donald Walsh

The Artist's Way
Julia Cameron

What Color is Your
Parachute?
Richard Nelson Bolles

The Seven Spiritual
Laws of Success
Deepak Chopra

A Book of Angels
Sophy Burnham

A Path with Heart
Jack Kornfield

The Prophet
Kahlil Gibran

Suppliers and further information

HEALTH AND BEAUTY
Alternative Therapies

Acupuncture
British Acupuncture Council
tel 020 8964 0222

Alexander Technique
Alexander Technique International
tel 020 7281 7639

Aromatherapy
International Federation of
Aromatherapists. Call for local
practitioners: 020 8742 2605

Biomagnetic Therapy
The British Biomagnetic Association
tel 01803 293 346

Chinese Herbal Medicine
Register of Chinese Herbal Medicine
tel 0208 904 1357

Chiropractic
The British Chiropractic Association
tel 01734 757 557

Colour Therapy
Hygeia College of Colour Therapy
tel 01453 832 150

Cranial Osteopathy
Cranial Osteopathic Association
tel 020 8367 5561

Crystal Healing
Affiliation of Crystal Healing
Organisations
tel 020 8398 7252

Feng Shui
Feng Shui Network International
tel 070 0033 6474
FengShuiNet.com

Flower Remedies
Dr Edward Bach Centre
tel 01491 834 678

Healing
National Federation of Spiritual Healers
Call for local practitioners:
tel 0891 616 080

Herbalists
General Council of Consultant Herbalists
Grosvenor House, 40 Sea Way
Middleton-on- Sea, West Sussex
PO22 7BA

Homeopathy
Society of Homeopaths
tel 01604 21400

Hypnotherapy
Central Register of Advanced
Hypnotherapists
tel 020 7359 6991

Light Therapy
SAD Association
t 01903 814 942

Massage
British Massage Therapy Council
tel 01772 881 063

Meditation
Transcendental Meditation
tel 0800 269 303

Reiki
www.reiki.org

Stress Management
International Stress Management
Association
Southbank University
103 Borough Road, London SE1 0AA
Write for local practitioners

Yoga
The British Wheel of Yoga
tel 01529 306 851

Bath Products

The Body Shop
tel 01903 733 888

Liberty's
tel 020 7734 1234

Lush
tel 020 7287 5874

Neal's Yard Natural Remedies
tel 020 7379 7222

Origins
tel 020 7823 6715

Cosmetics

Aveda
tel 020 7636 7911

Avon
tel 0800 663 664

Bobbi Brown Essentials
www.bobbibrown.com

Crabtree & Evelyn
tel 01235 862 244

Flori Roberts
tel 01279 421 555

Space NK
tel 020 7379 7030

MAC
tel 020 7349 0601

Clothing – accessories

Accessorize
tel 020 7240 2107

Lulu Guinness
tel 020 7823 4828

Paul Smith
tel 020 7836 7828

Clothing – basics
*indicates both ladies and menswear

Agnes B
tel 020 7225 3477

Benetton*
tel 020 7584 2563

Episode (Europe)
tel 020 7855 8500

French Connection*
tel 020 7399 7200

Gap*
tel 020 7287 3851
Hobbs
tel 020 836 0625
Jigsaw*
tel 020 7937 3572
Joseph
tel 020 7225 3335
Karen Millen
tel 020 7589 6459
Levi Strauss
tel 020 7292 2500
LK Bennett
tel 020 7376 7241
Max Mara
tel 020 7491 4748
Next* ✉
tel 845 600 7000
Oasis
tel 020 7452 1000
River Island Clothing*
tel 020 7499 3920
Warehouse
tel 020 7436 4179
Whistles
tel: 020 7487 4484
Zara
tel 020 7534 9500

Clothing – shoes
Bally
tel 020 7408 9877
LK Bennett
tel 020 7491 3005
Camper
tel 020 7379 8678
Lellio Bacio
tel 020 7224 4818
Natural Shoe Store
tel 020 7351 3721
Office
tel 020 7437 5275

Pied à Terre
tel 020 7376 0296
Russell & Bromley
tel 020 7589 8415

Clothing sizes

UK	US	French	Italian
10	6	40	44
12	8	42	46
14	10	44	48
16	12	46	50
18	14	48	52

Shoe sizes

UK	US	French	Italian
3	4.5	35	35
4	5.5	36	36
5	6.5	37	37
6	7.5	38	38
7	8.5	39	39
8	9.5	40	40

Health advice and products on the net
www.02simplify.com
www.allbeautyproducts.com
Listing of top beauty products.
www.auravita.com
www.body-herbals.com
www.boots.co.uk
www.emchealth.co.uk
Advice available on vitamins.
www.goodhealthdirectory.com
Advice on supplement and vitamins.
www.herbal-factory.mcmail.com
www.herbalnet.co.uk
www.health-shop.com
www.healthwb.co.uk
www.nutravida.co.uk
www.spellbound-online.co.uk
www.thisis.co.uk
Listing of alternative health associations.

Health and fitness
Contact your local leisure centre for details of local exercise classes and for recommended teachers.
David Lloyd Leisure Centres
For classes and sports courses.
tel 020 8446 8704
Salsa UK
For all events, classes and teachers.
www.salsa.co.uk

Healthy and organic food
Health4all
tel 01494 792789
www.health4all.co.uk
Goodness Direct
Wholefoods, organic products and herbal remedies straight to your door.
www.goodnessdirect.co.uk
Organics Direct
tel 020 7729 2828
Planet Organic
Organic produce by mail order.
tel 020 7221 1345
Simply Organic Food Ltd
tel 020 7622 5006
The Real Food Store
tel 020 7266 1162

Pets and pet products
Your local council will have a list of registered vets, boarding kennels and catteries in your area.
The Kennel Club
tel 0870 606 6700
The Feline Advisory Bureau
tel 01747 871872
www.vetscape.co.uk
Provides answers to pet owners' FAQs.
www.petplanet.co.uk
www.petspyjamas.co.uk
www.catsandcanines.com

HOME AND OFFICE

✉ denotes that mail order is available

For ease of use, the various items that might be required in the home and office have been categorised. Many of the recommended suppliers stock items that fall into many of the categories. These companies have been repeated where necessary, but their contact details only appear the first time that the company is listed. Please refer to the earlier listing for details.

Bedding

* indicates both beds and linens

The Conran Shop* ✉
tel 020 7589 7401
www.conran.co.uk

Descamps
tel 020 7235 6957

The General Trading Co
tel 020 7730 0411

Givan's Irish Linen
tel 020 7352 6352

Habitat*
tel 020 7631 3880
http://www.habitat.net

Harrods* ✉
tel 020 7730 1234

Harvey Nichols*
tel 020 7235 5000

Heals*
tel 020 7636 1666

The Iron Bed Company*
tel 020 7610 9903

John Lewis Partnership*
tel 020 7629 7711

Liberty* ✉
tel 020 7734 1234

Selfridges*
tel 020 7629 1234

Electrical

Argos*
tel 0870 600 2020

B&Q
tel 020 8591 7666

Comet
tel 020 8361 7999
http://www.comet.co.uk

Dixons
tel 020 7499 3494

Homebase
tel 020 8749 6982

House of Fraser*
tel 020 7963 2000

John Lewis Partnership
Details as before

Selfridges*
Details as before

Electrical goods suppliers on the net ✉

http://www.indexshop.com
http://www.electricaldiscount.co.uk
http://www.directelectricals.co.uk

Home and Office – Furniture and Stationery

Aero ✉
tel 020 7351 0511

Bureau
tel 020 7379 7898

The Conran Shop ✉
Details as before

Habitat
Details as before

Harrods ✉
Details as before

Heals
Details as before

The Holding Company ✉
tel 020 7352 1600
www.theholdingcompany.co.uk

Homebase
tel 020 8749 6982

Ikea UK Ltd
tel 020 8208 5600

Jerry's Home Store
tel 020 7581 0909

John Lewis Partnership
Details as before

Liberty ✉
Details as before

Muji
tel 020 7352 7148

Next ✉
tel 0845 600 7000

Ocean ✉
Home Shopping Catalogue
tel 020 7670 1234

Lighting

Aero ✉
Details as before

Babylon
tel 020 7376 7255

B&Q
Details as before

Christopher Wray Lighting
tel 020 7836 6869
www.christopher-wray.com

The Conran Shop ✉
Details as before

The General Trading Co
tel 020 7730 0411

Habitat
Details as before

Harrods ✉
Details as before

Heals
Details as before

Homebase
Details as before

Ikea UK Ltd
Details as before

John Lewis Partnership

Details as before

John Cullen Lighting

For contemporary design ideas.

tel 020 7371 5400

design@johncullenlighting.co.uk

Kensington Lighting Company

tel 020 7938 2405

Liberty ⊠

Details as before

Mr. Light

tel 020 7352 7525

Muji

Details as before

Selfridges ⊠

Details as before

SKK Lighting

tel 020 7434 4095

Paint

B&Q

Details as before

Farrow and Ball

tel 020 7351 0273

Habitat

Details as before

Homebase

Details as before

Ikea UK Ltd

Details as before

John Lewis Partnership

Details as before

John Oliver

tel 020 7221 6466

www.johnoliver.co.uk

Leyland SDM

tel 0800 454 484

www.leylandsdm.co.uk

Paint Service Co

They can match almost any colour.

tel 020 730 6408

Ray Munn Ltd.

tel 020 7493 9333

Selfridges ⊠

Details as before

Australian suppliers

Bedshed

Supply beds and bedlinen.

tel (08) 9242 2199

House & Garden

Locations in Burke, Brandon Park, Highpoint, Northland, Geelong, Shepparton, Albury, Wagga Wagga, Mackay, Bundaberg, Strathpine, Pacific Fair. See local directories for addresses and telephone listings.

Ikea

Locations in Gordon, Blacktown, Moore Park, Springwood, Moorabbin, Nunawading, Pert. See local directories for addresses and telephone listings.

KC Country Furniture

With stores in a number of locations, they supply quality furniture for home and office.

tel (02) 9907 0811

Canadian suppliers

Chapters Home and Garden Store ⊠

Everything for the home and garden, including kitchen equipment, linens, electrical appliances, gourmet foods and decorating tools and equipment.

www.chapters.ca

see also www.villa.ca

Heritage House Interiors, BC

Traditional and contemporary furniture.

(604) 946 2455

Villa Market Place

On-line listings for shops and mail order.

www.vmp.com

New Zealand suppliers

Courteneys Workshop

Specialists in children's furniture.

tel 09 524 0737

Elliot's Furniture Co Waili Ltd

Wood manufacturers of occasional furniture.

tel 07 863 8543

Hazelwoods

Quality furniture and furnishings available throughout New Zealand.

tel 04 528 2129

New Zealand's premier online office furniture stores

www.realdevelopments.net ⊠

www.netsynergy.co.nz ⊠

South African suppliers

Boardmans

tel (011)826 5151

Dursots ⊠

Food and drink on-line.

www.dursots.co.za

Hunkdory ⊠

On-line retail store specialising in unique products, mainly for children and babies, although they also supply linens, stationery and wine.

www.hunkydory.co.za

Stuttafords Stores

tel (011)616 2045

Sandton City

tel (011)783 5212

Traditional Furniture

Custom-built, handcrafted hardwood furniture for home and office.

www.traditionalfurniture.co.za

The Rosebank Mall

tel (011)788 1920

Westgate Shopping Mall

tel (011)768 1370

FOOD AND DRINK

⊠ denotes that mail order is available

Recipes and magazines

Bon Appetit

Monthly publication of Conde Nast/America.

www.epicurious.com

BBC Good Food

Monthly publication of BBC Worldwide Publishing.

Cooking Light

Monthly publication of Southern Progress Corp./America.

www.cookinglight.com

Gourmet

Monthly publication of Conde Nast/America.

Gourmet Traveller (Australia)

Monthly publication of Australian Consolidated Press.

Vogue Entertaining and Travel

Monthly publication of Conde Nast/Australia.

Waitrose Food Illustrated

Monthly publication of John Brown Contract Publishing.

Recipes found on the net

www.foodtv.com

www.world-of-recipes.com

www.cookinglight.com

www.globalgourmet.com

www.foodwine.com

Specialist foods

ASDA Superstores

tel 0113 243 5435

Bluebird

tel 020 7559 1222

Carluccio's

tel 020 7240 1487

Fortnum & Mason

tel 020 7734 8040

www.fortnumandmason.com

Harrods ⊠

tel 020 7730 1234

Harvey Nichols

tel 020 7584 0011

Luigis

tel 020 7352 7739

Planet Organic ⊠

tel 020 7727 8547

Sainsburys

tel 020 7695 6000

www.sainsburys.co.uk

Safeway

tel 020 8848 8744

Tesco

tel 020 8210 3600

www.tesco.co.uk

Waitrose

tel 020 8203 9711

www.waitrose.direct.com

Food shopping by net

www.botham.co.uk

www.cheesedirect.com

www.conran.co.uk

www.freshfood.co.uk

www.iorganic.com

www.organicsdirect.com

www.peck.it

Wines

Decanter Magazine

Monthly publication for enthusiasts.

www.decanter.com

Food and Wine

Information on good food and wine available on the net.

www.pathfinder.com/FoodWine

Oddbins ⊠

Information on champagne, wines, beers, spirits and special offers.

www.oddbins .com

One Minute Wine Expert

Quick tips on the web for finding the right wine for you.

www.winejournal.com

Quarterly Review of Wines

www.QRW.com

Vintage Wine Magazine

www.vintagewinemagazine.com

Winedine

British wine, restaurant and travel information on the web.

www.winedine.co.uk

Wine Enthusiast Magazine

14 Issues available per year.

www.wineenthusiastmag.com

winepros

www.winepros.com.au

Wine Spectator Magazine

www.winespectator.com

Wine Today

winetoday.com

Winestate Magazine

Information on Antipodean wines.

www.winestate.com.au

Wine X Magazine

www.winexwired.com

TRAVEL
Magazines

Travel and Leisure

Monthly publication by American Express.

www.travelandleisure.com

Conde Nast Traveller

Monthly publication from Conde Nast UK.

www.cntraveller.com

National Geographic

Monthly publication from National Geographic Society.

www.nationalgeographic.com

Australian Gourmet Traveller

Monthly publication from Australian Consolidated Press Limited.

www.gourmettraveller.com

Vogue Entertaining and Travel

Monthly publication of Conde Nast Australia.

Travel guides

Fodors Guides

Detailed guides for many countries.

www.fodors.com

Lonely Planet

Detailed guides for many countries.

www.lonelyplanet.com

Rough Guides

Guides for USA, Canada, Australia, Mexico, Hong Kong and India.

www.travel.roughguides.com

Dawsons Guides

Australian guides.

www.dawsons.com.au

Airlines

When travelling by air, call the airline before flying to check their baggage allowance, as it will change depending on the destination and your class of ticket. As a general guide take only one item of hand luggage and a maximum of one checked bag (no heavier than 32kg [70lbs]) on domestic flights and a maximum of two bags up to this weight on International flights

Aeroflot

www.aeroflot.org

Air Canada

www.aircanada.ca

Air France

www.airfrance.fr

British Airways

www.british-airways.com

British Midland

www.britishmidland.co.uk

Continental

www.continental.com

Delta

www.delta-air.com

Easy Jet

www.easyjet.co.uk

Go

www.go-fly.com

Northwest Airlines

www.nwa.com

Qantas

www.qantas.com.au

Ryanair

www.ryanair.com

South African Airways

www.saa.com

TWA

www.twa.com

Virgin Atlantic

virginatlantic.co.uk

Public transport

British Rail enquiries and reservations

tel 0845 7 48 49 50

Eurostar

www.eurostar.com

Eurotunnel

www.eurotunnel.com

On-line travel

On-line travel information and booking.

www.derby.ac.uk/library

Rail planner

www.rail.co.uk/uk rail/planner

The trainline

Information and booking of UK journeys.

www.thetrainline.com

Travelnet

Good deals on travel, including flights.

www.travelnet.co.uk

Uni-net

Uniting all travel networks throughout the country for up-to-date detailed information of all public transport.

www.uni-net.co.uk

London Transport information line

Information on trains, tubes and buses, and the best routes to your destination.

tel 020 72221234

For transport information in other cities call the local directory for details.

Checking by television

Travel Channel – Cable TV

Check your local listings for information.

www.travelchannel.com

CNN – Travel Guide

Check your local listings for information.

www.europe.cnn.com

Route planning

Streetmap UK

Streetmaps and ordnance survey maps available for the entire UK. It also gives the best road routes to your destination, approximate distance and travel time.

www.streetmap.co.uk

Streetmap USA

Highway trip-planning system that includes details of car hire and a cyber- router that will give you alternative routes to your destination and give approximate travel times. Also available are Citynet maps of many countries throughout the world.

Index

air travel 31, 35
  jet lag 34
  and packing 31, 32–33
alcohol, drinking 6, 139, *see* wines
aromatherapy oils 15, 47, 82

baking essentials 100
bank statements 72
baskets 82
bathing 130, 132–133
  and sleep 139, 142
bathrooms 9, 14–15, 58
  cleaning 14, 58, 61
bedrooms 9, 10, 24
  cleaning 59, 62
  see also beds; sleep
beds: books at bedtime 151
  mattresses and pillows 145
  sheets and duvet covers 146, 147
  things to do bedtime 11, 150
  things to keep next to 148
Beef Wrapped in Herbs (recipe) 108
belts 24
bills, dealing with 72
blood stains, removing 68
books: at bedtime 151
  getting rid of 71
breakfasts 9, 12

caffeine 13, 139
candles 82, 123, 130, 133
Caponata (recipe) 104
carbohydrate consumption 13
carpets: removing stains 68
cars: journeys 36
  pooling 28
cassettes, organising 75
CDs, organising 75
Cheese and Onion Spread
  (recipe) 104

children:
  amusing in cars 36
  and household chores 81
  and personal space 79, 85
  teaching to be tidy 59, 80
cleaning 57, 58, 59–63, 69
  stain removal 68, 69
clothes 9, 23
  and accessories 24
  bleaching 64
  dry cleaning 66
  drying 67
  ironing 64, 67
  organising 11, 18–21
  for travelling 32, 35
  washing 64, 66-67
colour, use of 10, 79, 86–87, 89
communal living 80–81
communication, effective 50–51
commuting 27, 28
condiments 100
cooking for guests *see* dinner
  parties
cooking utensils 98–99
Crab Quiche (recipe) 112
credit cards 72
cushions 82
cycling 28, 135

deadlines, meeting 49
decorating houses 10, 86–87, 89
dessert recipes 116
diaries: keeping 148
  sleep 140
dinner parties 95, 96, 102–103
  recipes 104–116
  wine 118-119
documents, important 72
dogs *see* pets
drinking/drinks 12, 100, 142
  see also alcohol; wines
dry cleaning 66

electrical cables, organising 75
emails 38, 39
exercise 6, 13, 28, 136
  aerobic 136
  cycling 28, 135
  games with friends 135, 137
  jogging 135, 137
  and sleep 139
  strength training 137
  walking 13, 28, 135
exfoliation 12, 133
eye make-up 16
eye masks 142

flowers and plants 42, 53, 82, 130
food 6, 13, 130
  and sleep 139, 142
fruit: for breakfast 12
  removing stains 68

gardening 135
goals, achieving 48–49, 52
grass stains, removing 68
grease stains, removing 68
guest rooms 95, 122–123
guests 95
  unexpected 57, 58
  see dinner parties; guest rooms
gum stains, removing 68

hair: accessories 24
  colour and make-up 16
  washing 11, 14
handbags 24
herbs 100
housework 57
  and children 81
  and communal living 80–81
  see cleaning; laundry

ink stains, removing 68
insomnia 139, 140

instruction manuals 72, 75
Internet 38–39, 41
    and home shopping 42–43
ironing 64, 67

jet lag 34
jewellery 24
jogging 135, 137

kitchens: cleaning 58, 63
    well-stocked 98–99, 100

lamps 82, 92
laundry 64, 66–67
Lebanese Soup, Chilled (recipe) 115
Lemon Chicken (recipe) 111
letters, old 71
light(ing) 15, 16, 46, 79, 126, 142
    artificial 82, 90-91, 92
lipstick: applying 16
    removing stains 68
living rooms 58, 82
    cleaning 60

mail-order shopping 42, 43
make-up, putting on 16
mattresses 145
meditation 6, 12, 126
moisturisers, using 14, 15, 16,
    132
music: organising CDs and tapes 75
    and sleep 143

newspapers, clearing out 71
nibbles (recipes) 104
notebooks, using 53, 54

offices see work/workplaces
oils, essential 15, 47, 82

packing 31, 32–33
painting 10, 86–87, 89

papers, dealing with 72
    see also newspapers
pasta 100
Pecan Puffs (recipe) 116
pets 36, 57, 76, 79, 126
photographs 71, 82
picnics 111, 120, 135
Pie Crust (recipe) 112
pillows 145
playrooms, children's 85
positivity 10, 51, 52, 143
pots and pans 98, 99

recycling 71
relaxation 9, 10, 14, 125, 126,
    129, 130–131; see also
    meditation
rice 100
rowing (boats) 135
rugs 82
    removing stains from 68

Salad, Overnight Lettuce (recipe) 106
shawls 24
shoes 23, 24
shopping, home: mail-order 42, 43
    on-line 42
showers 9, 12
sleep 10, 11, 130, 139, 140,
    142–143, 145
socks 23
Soufflé, Vegetable (recipe) 115
Soup, Chilled Lebanese (recipe) 115
spices 100
stains, removing 68, 69
starters 104
stress 6, 46–47, 48–49, 139;
see also relaxation
sugar, limiting 13
suitcases, packing 31, 32–33
Summer Fruit Cake (recipe) 116
swimming 135

throws 82
tidiness 9, 57, 58, 71, 72, 80–81
    teaching children 59, 80
travel 27
    and clothes 32, 35
    and packing 31, 32–33
    on public transport 27, 28
    weekends away 129
    see air travel; cars

underwear 11, 23

vacuum cleaners 69
Vegetable Soufflé, (recipe) 115
videos, organising 75
Vinaigrette (recipe) 107
visitors see guests
vitamin supplements 12

walking 13, 28, 135
wardrobes, organising 11, 18–21
warrantees 72
washing clothes 64–67
watches 24
weekends, relaxation 129
windows 92
wines 118–119
    and specific foods 96, 104, 106,
    107, 108, 111, 112, 115, 116
    stain removal 68
work/workplaces 45
    and communication 45, 50–51
    at home 45, 53
    and organisational skills 49, 52,
    54, 55
    and stress 46–47, 48
    things to do before leaving 55

yoga 137

Author's Acknowledgements

Saying thank you is such an important part of life. We don't say it often enough and it makes such a huge difference to how people around you feel. Do it more often! It really does feel good.

I have been truly blessed in my life to have so many people who have inspired me along the path. Each of them has taught me valuable lessons and has freely given their knowledge and love with open hearts. Many of their lessons have been passed on for you to share, and I hope they inspire you as they did me.

My husband, Jerry, has always given me the opportunity to be who I am and to enable me to fulfil my dreams. I have learned so very much about commitment and dedication to principles from him. They are most valuable lessons, as one should always keep their word in life. His love and faith in me even during difficult times are a reminder of how lucky I am. I'm sure I don't say thank you enough to him as we always take for granted the things and people that are closest to us.

This book would not have been possible without the time and commitment from all at Quadrille Publishing who produce such beautiful books. A very special thank you to Nicki Marshall, my editor, Anne Furniss for believing in the project, Helen Lewis for her great style and Coralie Bickford-Smith who worked on the layouts so enthusiastically.

I come from a long line of very strong women. My grandmother, Sarah, lived well into her nineties, and always told me that I was special; her strong belief in me encouraged me in all my creative endeavours. My mother, Mary, is now ninety and never ceases to amaze me with her insight into day-to-day living. I can only aspire to be so full of life when I reach her age. My sisters, Carol and Sue, encouraged me always to reach for the stars, another lesson that is worth remembering. My aunt, Lil, who passed away at 94 earlier this year, was a woman of great wisdom and great faith. She will always be a part of me.

I could not have written *How to do Everything and Still Have Time for Yourself* without the love, support, inspiration and wonderful sources of wisdom of my awesome friends – Andrew, for his beautiful pictures and spiritual insight; Judy Dobias, for her constant support and thirst for knowledge; Nina and Sergio, for their warmth and artistic passion; Tibye, one of my oldest and dearest friends whose spirituality is a constant source of comfort; Tessa and David, who make life seem like a wonderful adventure; Karen, whose strength and determination through adversity taught me the meaning of faith; Linda and Victor, who have seen me through some difficult times and whose cooking skills are unrivalled; Alison and Emma, my step-daughters, who keep me young and have taught me the true meaning of having a family; Beryl and Tim, who accepted a crazy American into their family and helped acclimatise me to the English way of life; Celia and Phil, who have shared in my business and creative development, offering all sorts of guidance along the way; Joannie, whose passion and sense of style are infectious; Jane, for her great Oz outlook on life; Sally O', who inspires me daily with her ability to create and motivate; Sandy Boler who sees the beauty in everything around her; Sarah, who taught me the gift of Reiki; Delacy who is a true healer and Kate, my guardian angel.

A special thank you to Amanda Skinner at John Amit Wines in London for her expertise in helping me to understand the world of wine. Cheers to you all.

Publishers' Acknowledgements and Picture Credits

All photographs in this book were taken by Andrew Wood and styled by Emily Jewsbury, with the exception of the following: 29 Magnum/Fernandino Scianna; 37 Gettyone Stone/Nicholas Parfitt; 40 Gettyone Stone/Luc Beziat; 65 DIAF/AlainLe Bot; 93 DIAF/H Gyssels; 121 Image Bank; 122 View/Peter Cook; 124 Photonica/Azu Oyama; 127 Gettyone Stone/James Darell; 134 Katz Pictures/Joe Pugliese/CPi, 1998; 141 Magnum/Leonard Freed. Photographs on pages 1, 14, 17, 18, 44, 48, 53, 56, 59, 74, 101, 128, 131, 132, 149 and 150 were taken by Andrew Wood for The Holding Company. Our thanks to everyone at Camron PR for their help in securing these images. Our thanks go to Sania Pell and Jake Harley for appearing in the photographs and to Couveture, based on the King's Road in London, who supplied the bed linen.